Wholesome

Low Cholesterol Cookbook

2,000 Days of Delicious Heart-Healthy Recipes, Featuring a 30-Day Meal Plan for Optimal Cardiovascular Health

Debra Lincoln

Copyright © 2024 by Debra Lincoln

All rights reserved. No part of this book may be copied, shared, or transmitted by any means, whether electronic or mechanical, without the publisher's prior written permission. Exceptions include brief quotations used in critical reviews and other non-commercial uses allowed by copyright law.

Contents

- Acknowledgments
- About The Author
- Lisa's Journey to Reducing Her Cholesterol Levels

SECTION 1

- What is cholesterol?
- Types of Cholesterol
- Factors Influencing Cholesterol Level
- Lowering your Cholesterol Through your Diet
- Embracing Healthier Living

RECIPES

Breakfast

- Chocolate Pancakes
- Cinnamon Granola
- Hot Pepper and Salsa Frittata
- Peach and Raspberry Soufflé
- Slow-cooker fruity Oatmeal
- Apple Pie Spice Soufflé
- Berry-Infused French Toast Delight
- Protein-rich buckwheat Pancakes

Contents

- Blueberry-Banana Smoothie
- Blueberry-Banana Smoothie
- PB&J Smoothies
- Nutritious Oat-Nut Trail Bars

Bread and muffins

- Zucchini Nut Loaf
- Cinnamon Hazelnut Pastries
- Berry-Oat Coffee Cake
- Carrot-Oat Loaf
- Apple-Cranberry Nut Loaf
- Morning Delight Muffins
- Savory Cheddar and Herb Biscuits
- Hearty Whole-Grain Cornbread
- Oat-bran and Date Muffins
- Aromatic Pumpkin Bread

Poultry

- Chicken Breasts with Salsa
- Asian Chicken Stir-Fry
- Mashed Bean-Topped Chicken Breasts
- New Potatoes with Chicken Breasts
- Tomato Sauce Poached Chicken
- Hazelnut-Crusted Chicken Breasts

Contents

- Turkey Stuffed with Prune
- Texas BBQ Chicken Thighs
- Turkey Cutlets Florentine
- Turkey Cutlets Parmesan
- Chicken Pesto with Hazelnuts
- Chilled Chicken with Cherry Tomato Sauce

Salads

- Charred Petite Beet Medley Salad
- Crisp Jicama and Red Lettuce Salad
- Warm New Potato Salad
- Hearty Wheat Berry Salad
- Pasta Salad with Crisp Vegetables
- French-Style Lentil Rice Salad
- Low-Fat Red Bean Salad with Taco Chips
- Crab and Edamame Salad with Surimi
- Apple Coleslaw
- Citrus Salad
- Black-Eyed Pea Salad

Vegetables

- Oven-Roasted Citrus Beets
- Sautéed Ginger Sugar-Snap Peas
- Crispy Fried Green Tomatoes

Contents

- Herb-crusted Baby Eggplants
- Snow Peas with Shallots
- Buttermilk Mashed Potatoes
- Grilled Corn with Red Peppers
- Oven-Roasted Garlic Corn
- Cheesy Polenta
- Chilled Veggie-Stuffed Tomatoes
- Baked Tomatoes with Garlic
- Farro Pilaf

Appetizer snacks and beverages

- Spicy Roasted Red Bell Pepper Dip
- Vanilla and Sweet Spice Dip with Dried Plums and Pecans
- Fresh Basil and Kalamata Hummus
- Zucchini Spread
- Nectarine-Plum Chutney
- Canapés with Roasted Garlic, Artichoke, and Chèvre Spread
- Stuffed Cremini Mushrooms with Kale and Ham
- Orange-Strawberry Drink
- Pineapple Bliss Shake
- Banana Mini Snack Cakes

Contents

Soups

- Hearty Barley Vegetable Soup
- Simple Parmesan Pasta Soup
- Cajun Gumbo with Greens and Ham
- Creamy Broccoli-Cheese Soup
- Tomato Soup with Pasta and Chickpeas
- Three-Pepper and Bean soup with Rotini
- Zesty Spinach Soup with a Lemon Twist

Fish and Seafood

- Fish Fillets with Roasted-Veggie Rice
- Hearty Fish Chowder
- Crunchy Italian Catfish
- Grilled Cod with a Creamy Artichoke and Horseradish Sauce
- Oven-Baked Flounder with Tomato Crust
- Asian-Style Poached Halibut with Broth
- Broiled Salmon with Black Olive Pesto
- Grilled Salmon with Mediterranean Flavors
- Pan-Seared Salmon with Broccoli and Brown Rice
- Rotini with Smoky Chipotle Salmon Cream
- Tilapia with Lemon-Crumb Topping
- Trout with Almonds and Orange-Dijon Yogurt Sauce

Contents

Meat

- Teriyaki-Style Grilled Sirloin
- Balsamic-braised beef with Assorted Mushrooms
- Sirloin Steak with Portobello Mushrooms
- Slow-Cooker Pepper Steak
- Bulgur and Lean Beef Bake
- Hawaiian Meatballs
- Southwestern Beef-Stuffed Pita Tacos
- Bean-Enriched Bunless Beef Burger
- Pork Tenderloin with Refined Sauce

Dessert

- Pumpkin-Carrot Cake
- Chocolate Mini-Cheesecakes
- Fresh Peach and Ginger Crisp
- Light Baklava
- Chocolate Soufflés with Vanilla Sauce
- Strawberry Margarita Ice

Bonus

Exercising

- Basic Aerobic Training

Contents

- Increasing Flexibility: Crucial Stretches
- Tips for sticking with your exercise plans

Worksheets

- **Grocery Shopping worksheet**
- **Weekly Fitness worksheet**

Acknowledgments

I am deeply thankful to many individuals for their contributions to this work:

I extend my heartfelt gratitude to my husband, Stephen Lincoln, whose unwavering encouragement and support played a crucial role in bringing this dream to life. His words resonated with me, and his assistance was invaluable in addressing the technical challenges encountered during the book's formatting process.

I am profoundly grateful to Amelia Richards, a highly respected medical doctor and dear friend, who graciously took the time to meticulously review every line of this manuscript, despite her demanding responsibilities with her family and medical practice.

My sincere thanks go out for the enduring friendships and the immense support I have received throughout this journey.

About The Author

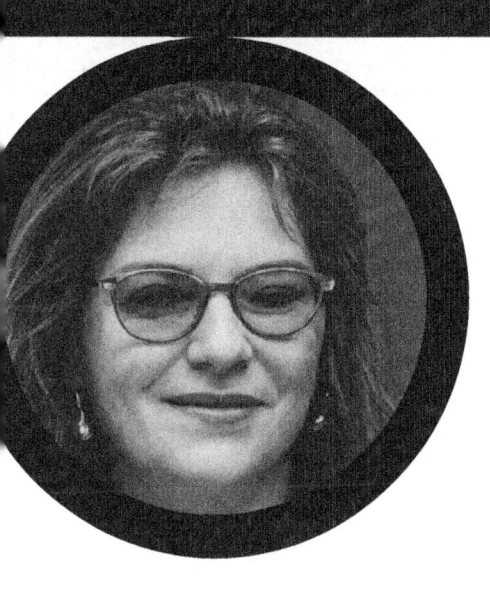

Dr. Debra Lincoln is a dedicated advocate for holistic healthcare and natural medicine. As a certified medical doctor with years of experience, she combines traditional medicine with contemporary scientific knowledge. Based in the UK, Dr. Debra has committed her career to helping individuals improve their well-being through natural methods.

Beyond her clinical practice, Dr. Debra actively promotes healthier living by conducting regular workshops and seminars as an enthusiastic educator. She also writes articles on herbal remedies, health topics, and holistic wellness for various magazines and has authored several books on these subjects.

Dr. Debra values spending time with her family. She and her husband, Stephen Lincoln, who shares her passion for natural lifestyles, enjoy exploring nature, gardening, and experimenting with medicinal plants in their home lab.

Lisa's Journey to Reducing Her Cholesterol Levels

I'm Lisa, a 58-year-old cisgender woman, and I was quite concerned when a routine check-up revealed my cholesterol level was 300 mg/dl. It was surprising, given my commitment to a healthy lifestyle, which includes a predominantly organic vegetarian Mediterranean-based diet, regular yoga, Pilates, and meditation. I decided against pharmaceutical treatments and sought natural methods to address the root cause of my high cholesterol.

The initial nutrient analysis showed that while most vitamins and minerals in my diet were sufficient, I was low in total energy, carbohydrates, proteins, phosphorus, calcium, potassium, copper, and iodine. Additionally, my diet lacked CoQ10-rich foods like oily fish, and my omega-3 intake was insufficient. I also tended to drink alcohol three or four times a week when dining out.

I have always had high cholesterol since my early twenties, and it had recently spiked to dangerous levels. Despite this, my ASCVD risk was a low 2.0%, although it was slightly above the optimal range. My goal was to lower my total and LDL cholesterol through dietary adjustments to reduce my 10-year ASCVD risk.

Working with my nutritionist Dr. Debra Lincoln, she developed a personalized meal plan that increased my fiber intake while decreasing the glycemic index of my foods. She also increased my protein and omega-3 consumption. To boost my fiber intake, I added more nuts and seeds and included an extra serving of fruit each day.

I also incorporated more high-intensity interval training (HIIT) workouts suggested by Dr. Debra Lincoln into my exercise regimen to enhance bone health and raise my HDL cholesterol. Additionally, resistance training was included to lower total and LDL cholesterol levels.

After five months of these changes, my numbers improved significantly: my total cholesterol dropped by 83 points, LDL decreased by 62 points, VLDL reduced by 7 points, and triglycerides fell by 34 points. My ASCVD risk also dropped from 2.0% to 1.7%, surpassing the optimal target.

This journey shows how a complete change in nutrition and lifestyle can naturally lower cholesterol levels and improve cardiovascular health. I am forever grateful to Dr. Debra Lincoln.

You are welcome!

Dear Reader,

Thank you for selecting this Low Cholesterol Cookbook as your guide towards better well-being.

This book has been structured to help you control your cholesterol levels naturally. It contains nutrition information, delicious heart-healthy recipes, and a step-by-step meal plan for you.

We hope you find this book both inspiring and practical. May these recipes and lifestyle tips lead you to healthier cholesterol levels.

Wishing you good health and happiness,

My sincere thanks,
Dr Debra Lincoln.

Debra Lincoln

Your Bonus

We're excited to offer you a special bonus! Scan the QR code below to claim your free bonus cookbook. As a bonus, you'll also gain access to our exclusive cookbook community, where you can ask questions, share tips, and connect with our team. Don't miss out—just scan the QR code below to get started!

Enjoy and happy cooking!

Important Notice

Dear Reader,

We understand that our Low Cholesterol Cookbook will be used by individuals worldwide, and that units of measurement can vary—such as ounces in the U.S. and grams in the U.K.

To assist you with conversions, we've provided a link to a measurement calculator website below. This tool will be invaluable in converting any cooking measurements in this cookbook to your preferred units.

Simply scan the QR code below

- What is cholesterol?
- Types of Cholesterol
- Factors Influencing Cholesterol Level
- Lowering your Cholesterol Through your Diet
- Embracing Healthier Living

Section 1

What is cholesterol?
why should you care about it?

Only one aspect of the fight against heart disease is cholesterol levels. The battle against heart disease happens to be cholesterol, which is the leading cause of death in the world. But it's a factor you can control by changing your diet, eating healthier foods, and exercising more often. If you follow the instructions in this cookbook within months you will make small changes that will add up to big improvements for your health.

What Is Cholesterol?

Cholesterol is a fatty substance produced by the liver from two acetate molecules. It is only found in animals. Cholesterol helps produce hormones and steroids, and it is also an important component of cell membranes. We need some amount of cholesterol for our bodies to function properly, but having too much or too little can signal problems such as atherosclerosis (clogged arteries), heart attack, or stroke. Certain types of cholesterol may increase disease risk more than others depending on how they interact with other substances in the body.

For cholesterol to travel within the bloodstream, it must attach itself to proteins and fats, forming complexes called lipoproteins. These lipoproteins occur as **High-density (HDL) lipoproteins and Low-density (LDL) lipoproteins.**

Total cholesterol levels up to 200 mg/dL are generally considered normal;

however, your health status or risk factors might necessitate your doctor advising differently depending on your circumstances. Levels between 200-239 mg/dL require assessment for the LDL/HDL ratio.

Cholesterol levels vary due to genetics, age, and sex, usually increasing with age. Men often have higher levels than premenopausal women, but this trend changes upon reaching menopause for most females.

HDL Cholesterol

High-density lipoprotein (HDL) is sometimes referred to as "good" cholesterol because it helps remove LDL cholesterol from the bloodstream, sending it back to the liver where it gets processed and eliminated from the body. It acts like a detergent in arteries because, according to studies, high HDL levels lower LDL cholesterol and make it difficult for atheroma or plaque formation inside arterial walls. Foods such as olives, nuts, avocados, peanut butter, whole grain cereals, and other fiber-rich items; moderate alcohol consumption; dried beans and peas; fish; and citrus fruits like oranges and tangerines can increase HDL levels. An HDL value of more than 40 mg/dL is essential for good health and can be influenced significantly by diet and exercise.

LDL Cholesterol

LDL is often called "bad" cholesterol because low-density lipoprotein (LDL) carries cholesterol from the liver to the bloodstream, creating plaques in arteries. Oatmeal, orange juice, apples, nuts, flaxseed or linseed oil, fatty fish like salmon or sardines, legumes like lentils or chickpeas, barley, cherries, and vegetables are all examples of foods that help lower LDL levels. The ideal range for LDL is less than 100 mg/dL, while over 160 mg/dL is considered high. Dietary control of fat intake along with physical activity helps manage levels of LDL in our bodies.

Total/HDL Cholesterol Ratio

The total cholesterol over HDL ratio predicts the risk of heart disease. It's calculated by dividing the total cholesterol level by the HDL level. You want the result to be below 3.5 to 1; a ratio above 5 to 1 shows a high risk for heart diseases.

Factors Influencing Cholesterol level

Other fats, hormones, and molecules within the blood may lead to variations in heart disease risks. These factors can be assessed using a comprehensive blood test panel. Additional factors such as these might be tested for when there exist several underlying risk factors for cardiovascular diseases. you should consult a physician about testing if you fall under these categories.

Triglycerides

The fats in the bloodstream are called triglycerides. When you consume more calories than your body needs, the extra calories are turned into triglycerides and stored in fat cells. A diet high in carbohydrates or simple sugars can increase triglyceride levels. People with high amounts of these fats often also have high cholesterol levels, putting them at greater risk for heart disease. A person is considered to have normal levels if they are at or below 150 mg/dL based on a fasting blood test.

Homocysteine

Homocysteine is an amino acid produced by the body from meat when there is not enough B vitamin. When levels are high, it can damage the walls of arteries, increasing the chance of a blood clot forming. Foods high in folate, such as whole grain cereals, oranges, broccoli, beetroot, nuts, etc., may help reduce homocysteine levels. Vitamin supplements containing folic acid (a synthetic form) are also recommended.

Genetic Factors

Some blood compounds, such as VLDL and Lp(a) cholesterol, can be entirely genetic, which means they cannot be controlled with diet and exercise alone. Very low-density lipoprotein (VLDL) cholesterol is a form of LDL that contains a lot of triglyceride, while Lp(a) is just a different type of LDL cholesterol that carries much greater risks for coronary artery disease. If any of these compounds are found in your body, seek medical help right away for suitable drugs.

Lowering your Cholesterol Through your Diet

One good strategy to take care of our hearts is understanding nutrition basics and then incorporating them into our daily lives consistently. This knowledge will enable us to come up with creative recipes for cooking healthy foods meant for the heart. Lowering one's cholesterol even slightly has been shown to greatly improve overall health, as a minor decrease in its levels by 1% leads to an equally lower chance of getting heart disease by 2%, thus serving as an incentive to stick to this type of plan

Essentials for Healthy Eating

When planning your meals at home or selecting food when dining out, the key is to maintain a well-balanced diet that includes a variety of food groups. If you find yourself overindulging in certain foods one day, balance it out by consuming less of those foods in the subsequent days. You can still enjoy your favorite foods while ensuring you meet the nutritional requirements for a healthy diet and limit less healthy options.

Basic Nutrition Guidelines for a Healthy Diet

➤ **Whole Grains:** Ensure at least half of your grain intake consists of whole grains.

➤ **Low-Fat Dairy:** Include fat-free or low-fat dairy products.

➡ **Omega-3 Rich Fish:** Eat fish high in omega-3 fatty acids at least twice a week.

➡ **Lean Meats and Poultry:** Choose lean meats and poultry without skin, and prepare them without adding saturated and trans fats.

➡ **Healthy Fats:** Limit saturated and trans fats, and opt for monounsaturated and polyunsaturated fats instead.

➡ **Low Salt and Sugar:** Choose foods with little or no added salt and reduce the consumption of sugary foods and beverages.

Fruits and Vegetables

Vegetables and fruits are nutrient-dense and low in calories, providing essential vitamins, minerals, fiber, and other nutrients. Aim to eat a colorful variety, such as green spinach, red tomatoes, and orange carrots, to maximize nutritional benefits.

➡ **Healthy Hints**

- Opt for canned vegetables and beans labeled no-salt-added or low sodium. Manufacturers are increasingly offering healthier options.

- For canned fruits, look for products with minimal added sugar. Fruits canned in water have fewer calories compared to those in juice or syrup. Rinsed and drained cans reduce the number of these substances even further.

Grains

Grains include foods made from wheat, rice, oats, corn, and other cereals such as bread, pasta, oatmeal, and grits. There are two categories: whole grains and refined grains. Aim to make at least half of your grain consumption whole grains because they are richer in fiber and complex carbohydrates and lower in saturated fat compared to refined grains. Whole grains contain the entire grain kernel–the bran, germ, and endosperm. Healthy options include whole-wheat flour, oatmeal, brown rice, quinoa, and whole-grain cereals and bread. Refined grains have been milled, removing the bran and germ, and some fiber, B vitamins, and iron. Although most enriched grains add back some B vitamins and iron, fiber is not restored. Examples of enriched grains are white rice, and wheat flour-enriched bread.

Healthy Hints

- To find whole grains, read the ingredients list beyond the packaging labels. Choose products where the whole grain is listed first.

- Avoid commercial baked goods such as muffins, cakes, pies, and cookies, which typically consist of refined grains and contain large amounts of calories and fewer nutrients. Make your own at home with whole wheat flour, unsaturated oils, fruits, and vegetables for healthier snacks.

Dairy Products

Dairy products are essential in healthy eating patterns because they supply necessary protein as well as calcium. For instance, adults aged 19 to 50 should take in 1,000 milligrams of calcium daily, while those aged 51 years or more require about 1,200 milligrams. Saturated fat consumption can be reduced by using fat-free or low-fat dairy products. Healthy options include cream cheese, yogurt, milk (fat-free or low-fat), sour cream, and cheese. You may also compare nutrition labels to find products with less saturated fat and calories.

> **Healthy Hints**
>
> - Many cheeses are very high in sodium and fat content. Fat-free or low-fat alternatives may contain excessive sugar levels too. Please look over nutrition labels before buying any product.
>
> - Gradually reduce the amount of whole milk you drink to make the move easier.
>
> - If you don't use dairy products, there are good sources of calcium available like legumes, soybean foods, and green leafy vegetables such as spinach, kale, and broccoli.

Fish and Seafood

Research shows that eating oily fish high in omega-3 fatty acids, such as salmon, herring, sardines, mackerel, and albacore tuna, can reduce the risk of heart disease. Include at least two servings of these types of fish in your diet every week. Fish oil supplements may be recommended for people with heart disease or high triglyceride levels by healthcare providers to boost their intake of omega-3 fats. Shrimp, squid, scallops, mussels, and clams are examples of shellfish with low levels of saturated fat, which also provide protein for a healthy heart.

> **Healthy Hints**
>
> - Canned tuna is a great source of omega-3s. Go for low-sodium varieties canned in water or vacuum-sealed pouches.
>
> - However, all fish and shellfish may contain traces of mercury or other contaminants; these health risks depend on the kind of fish and the quantity consumed. By combining various kinds, you prevent being particularly vulnerable to negative impacts. Tilefish, shark, swordfish, and king mackerel should be avoided by pregnant women or those planning a pregnancy because they have large amounts of mercury according to FDA advice. The advantages of eating fish outweigh the disadvantages.
>
> - Low-sodium, low-fat seasonings like herbs, spices, and lemon juice are good for cooking fish.

Poultry and Meat

Lean poultry (meat) without the skin is an excellent source of protein that helps you feel full longer and maintains muscle strength, especially during the aging process. For instance, it is said you should not eat more than 6 ounces per day of cooked lean skinless poultry or lean meat. These include skinless chicken/turkey breasts, lean beef cuts like round steak, sirloin, and rump roast, extra lean ground beef, lean pork loin chops and tenderloin.

> **Healthy Hints**

- Choose whole turkeys or turkey breasts without added fat or broth.
- Go for the USDA Select grades of meat as they have less marbling than Prime or Choice cuts.
- Remove any visible fats before cooking.
- Poultry and meat lose 25% of their weight after being cooked, e.g. 4 ounces of raw meat equals about 3 ounces cooked.
- Cool meat juices and skim off solidified fat for healthier sauces, stews, and soups.
- Minimize your intake of processed meats such as bacon and sausages due to high levels of saturated fats and sodium. Look out for low-calorie, low-saturated fat, low-sodium brands when choosing reduced-fat varieties.

Sodium

Salt shaker alone is not responsible for most dietary sodium content; this comes from packaged as well as processed foodstuffs. Most dietary sodium comes from packaged foods rather than salt shakers. Above-normal amounts of sodium may lead to hypertension. For blood pressure control, try consuming less than 2400 mg per day if possible. Reducing it to about 1500 mg will give more advantages.

> **Healthy Hints**

- Lowest-sodium-content products should always be selected based on nutritional labeling found on food items available at stores

- When preparing food at home you can use salt-free seasonings and flavorings that include herbs, spices, and lemon or lime juice.

- Before going to a restaurant, look over the menu online and choose items that are not sodium-laden.

Fats and Oils

It is the type of fat that you consume rather than the amount that affects your blood cholesterol. Saturated fats, trans fats, and unsaturated fats are three major kinds found in food. Try to limit the intake of saturated fatty acids to less than 5-6% of total calories per day; minimize the consumption of foods with trans-fatty acids. you should take less than 13 grams daily. The content of saturated fat can be obtained from nutritional information provided on most packages throughout food stores.

Choose better options like polyunsaturated or monounsaturated fats contained in liquid vegetable oils, nuts, seeds (flaxseed), and fish such as salmon and mackerel among others such oils include canola oil, olive oil, or soybean oil; mayonnaise dressings prepared from these should also be chosen instead. Essentially this means:

UNSATURATED OILS: Opt for slightly salted) or light margarine made from unsaturated oils. Available choices include Canola; Olive; and

29

Soybean oil.

SOFT MARGARINES: These can be easily categorized into two types: margarines with unsaturated vegetable oil as the first ingredient and those containing hydrogenated oils. The optimum intake level is equivalent to four (4) servings or a single serving which is equal to 2 ounces and very limited amounts of fats and sweets.

NUTS AND SEEDS: However, since they are high in calories, eat them sparingly because they contain beneficial fats.

OILY FISH: For instance, salmon and mackerel; are rich in fat that is good for your health.

When saturated fats are solid at room temperature while liquid ones are more healthy. Avoid trans-fats by using only liquid vegetable oils or trans-fat-free soft margarine instead of solid fats like butter.

> ### ▶ Healthy Hints
>
> - Select products labeled "low in saturated fat".
>
> - Use soft margarine or liquid/melted ones when cooking and flavoring foods, but not while baking - your pastries may become too watery due to added water.
>
> - The healthiest option would be cooking sprays instead of butter or oil – compatibility has to be checked with cookware.
>
> - Be attentive to trans-fat on the nutrition facts panel but do not forget

- about saturated fat levels." Trans-fat-free" does not mean low in saturated fat.

Added Sugars

Differentiate between sugars found in fruits and milk from those that are added during food processing. On the other hand, added sugars have no nutrients but contribute to overweight and reduced heart health. We advise restricting added sugars to less than half of your discretionary calorie allowance per day.

➡ Healthy Hints

- Gradually reduce the amount of sugar you add to foods and drinks.

- Find replacements for sugary drinks such as sugar-free or low-calorie varieties, a splash of citrus fruit, or plain water.

- Go for fruits instead of sweets, choose those canned in water or natural juice, and drain off extra syrup or juice.

- Cut down on sugar in recipes by using extracts or cinnamon for the sweet taste instead of sugar.

Embracing Healthier Living

It is simple: Regular exercise is a powerful prevention against heart-related diseases; it reduces cholesterol levels, and blood pressure thus helping in weight loss. In addition to becoming healthier physically, you may find yourself not only feeling better but also having more energy and being able to make further positive lifestyle changes with greater ease.

Maintain Activity Levels

For optimum heart health, we recommend at least 120 minutes of moderate-intensity exercise or at least 85 minutes per week of vigorous-intensity exercise supplemented with muscle-strengthening activities at least twice weekly. Aim for an easy 30-minute session every day for four days a week. If you want to lower your pressure and cholesterol, aim for an average of 40 minutes about three times a week. That can be anything from moderate to vigorous aerobic activity.

Feel free to break up your exercise into chunks ten minutes long or longer throughout each day including some moderate activities like gardening and housework which will all together add up towards your daily physical activity account

Take this chart into account when estimating how many calories are burned during various activities performed at different intensities (see table below).

Remember that factors such as sex, current weight, and muscle mass affect calorie consumption. The figures provided are for a 160-pound person; so if you weigh less than this, the rate of calorie burn will be different.

Activity	Calories Burned within 30 minutes
Dancing	172
Walking (5 mph)	155
Aerobics	250
Bicycling	150
Basketball	198
Stretching	75
Hiking	190
Swimming	270

If you have not been active, had a heart attack, or have conditions such as high blood pressure, high cholesterol, diabetes, obesity, or smoking cigarettes, consult with your healthcare professional before starting a new exercise program. Additionally, consider it if you are over sixty-five years old or if heart disease is running in your family.

Weight Management

Understanding and changing habits that hinder effective weight management is essential for adopting healthier behaviors and ensuring a longer, more robust life. Keep in mind that age can cause caloric needs to decrease even when activity level remains unchanged so calculate your ideal daily intake based on age, gender, and activity level.

Balance Your Caloric Intake

To avoid piling up more pounds than what you already have today you must ensure that your calories from all sources do not exceed those burned daily. This has nothing to do with eating unnecessarily stomachful meals but in reality, every time these requirement levels are exceeded then weight gain commences gradually.

Know When To Lose Weight

Even without other risk factors, carrying excess weight significantly increases your risk of heart disease and stroke. Possessing too much body weight can lead to lower levels of good HDL cholesterol and higher levels of bad LDL cholesterol in overweight people. Pay attention to how fat is distributed in your body as that could tell your level of risk. Having a waist measurement above 40 inches for men or 35 inches for women puts them at increased risk. Even losing only a small amount of total body weight can improve blood cholesterol profiles.

Check the Body Mass Index (BMI) to know which category you fall into. This technique uses both your height and body mass. If you have a BMI that classifies you as obese or overweight with additional risk factors, consult with your healthcare provider about setting a healthy weight goal for yourself. If you are normally weighted or overweight but without any other risks, do not worry about losing weight; make sure instead that it remains constant. Control your weight effectively by taking in the right number of calories and participating in regular physical exercise.

To calculate BMI, weigh yourself without clothes or shoes on while measuring your height. **Next, find where your height is plotted on the chart after scanning the QR code below and locate what range you belong to.**

Do Not Smoke and Avoid Secondhand Smoke

If you are a Smoker, you should consult your physicians on the most effective ways to quit smoking. By quitting smoking, you significantly reduce your chance of heart disease or stroke

Moderate Drinking

Even though consuming alcohol moderately has been associated with lowered chances of heart disease, you should drink responsibly. Females are expected to consume not more than a single glass each day while males can gulp down two. Overindulgence in alcohol may lead to various grave health problems such as hypertension, congestive heart failure, and increased calorie intake minus nutrition value. If you want to consume alcohol, do it within limits; but if you don't take it now, there is no need to start.

30 Day Meal Plan

Week 1

Days	Breakfast	Lunch	Snack	Dinner
01	Zucchini Spread with Whole Wheat Pita	Chicken Breasts with Salsa	Zucchini Nut Loaf	Fish Fillets with Roasted-Veggie Rice
02	Cinnamon Granola	Charred Petite Beet Medley Salad	Morning Delight Muffins	Asian Chicken Stir-Fry
03	Hot Pepper and Salsa Frittata	Warm New Potato Salad	Aromatic Pumpkin Bread	Grilled Cod with a Creamy Artichoke and Horseradish Sauce
04	Peach and Raspberry Soufflé	Turkey Cutlets Florentine	Savory Cheddar and Herb Biscuits	Broiled Salmon with Black Olive Pesto
05	Slow-Cooker Fruity Oatmeal	French-Style Lentil Rice Salad	Hearty Whole-Grain Cornbread	Teriyaki-Style Grilled Sirloin
06	Apple Pie Spice Soufflé	Low-Fat Red Bean Salad with Taco Chips	Oat-bran and Date Muffins	Oven-Baked Flounder with Tomato Crust
07	Berry-Infused French Toast Delight	Hearty Wheat Berry Salad	Morning Delight Muffins	Slow-Cooker Pepper Steak

Week 2

Days	Breakfast	Lunch	Snack	Dinner
08	Protein-rich Buckwheat Pancakes	Apple Coleslaw	Stuffed Cremini Mushrooms with Kale and Ham	Pan-Seared Salmon with Broccoli and Brown Rice
09	Spicy Roasted Red Bell Pepper Dip with Veggie Sticks	Crab and Edamame Salad with Surimi	Light Baklava	Turkey Cutlets Parmesan
10	Nutritious Oat-Nut Trail Bars	Citrus Salad	Chocolate Soufflés with Vanilla Sauce	Grilled Salmon with Mediterranean Flavors
11	Chocolate Pancakes	Hearty Barley Vegetable Soup	Zucchini Spread with Whole Grain Crackers	Trout with Almonds and Orange-Dijon Yogurt Sauce
12	Cinnamon Granola	Crisp Jicama and Red Lettuce Salad	Fresh Basil and Kalamata Hummus with Veggie Sticks	Hawaiian Meatballs
13	Hot Pepper and Salsa Frittata	Tomato Soup with Pasta and Chickpeas	Oat-bran and Date Muffins	Tilapia with Lemon-Crumb Topping
14	Peach and Raspberry Soufflé	Black-Eyed Pea Salad	Savory Cheddar and Herb Biscuits	Sirloin Steak with Portobello Mushrooms

Week 3

Days	Breakfast	Lunch	Snack	Dinner
15	Protein-rich Buckwheat Pancakes	Stuffed Cremini Mushrooms with Kale and Ham	Aromatic Pumpkin Bread	Pan-Seared Salmon with Broccoli and Brown Rice
16	PB&J Smoothies	Crab and Edamame Salad with Surimi	Carrot-Oat Loaf	Turkey Cutlets Parmesan
17	Nutritious Oat-Nut Trail Bars	Citrus Salad	Chocolate Soufflés with Vanilla Sauce	Grilled Salmon with Mediterranean Flavors
18	Chocolate Pancakes	Hearty Barley Vegetable Soup	Zucchini Spread with Whole Grain Crackers	Trout with Almonds and Orange-Dijon Yogurt Sauce
19	Pumpkin-Carrot Cake	Crisp Jicama and Red Lettuce Salad	Hearty Whole-Grain Cornbread	Hawaiian Meatballs
20	Vanilla and Sweet Spice Dip with Dried Plums and Pecans	Tomato Soup with Pasta and Chickpeas	Oat-bran and Date Muffins	Tilapia with Lemon-Crumb Topping
21	Peach and Raspberry Soufflé	Black-Eyed Pea Salad	Orange-Strawberry Drink	Sirloin Steak with Portobello Mushrooms

40

Week 4

Days	Breakfast	Lunch	Snack	Dinner
22	Slow-Cooker Fruity Oatmeal	Low-Fat Red Bean Salad with Taco Chips	Carrot-Oat Loaf	Grilled Salmon with Mediterranean Flavors
23	PB&J Smoothies	French-Style Lentil Rice Salad	Chocolate Soufflés with Vanilla Sauce	Teriyaki-Style Grilled Sirloin
24	Canapés with Roasted Garlic, Artichoke, and Chèvre Spread	Citrus Salad	Fresh Peach and Ginger Crisp	Grilled Salmon with Mediterranean Flavors
25	Protein-rich Buckwheat Pancakes	Apple Coleslaw	Stuffed Cremini Mushrooms with Kale and Ham	Pan-Seared Salmon with Broccoli and Brown Rice
26	Pumpkin-Carrot Cake	Crisp Jicama and Red Lettuce Salad	Hearty Whole-Grain Cornbread	Hawaiian Meatballs
27	Nutritious Oat-Nut Trail Bars	Citrus Salad	Berry-Oat Coffee Cake	Grilled Salmon with Mediterranean Flavors
28	Peach and Raspberry Soufflé	Black-Eyed Pea Salad	Orange-Strawberry Drink	Sirloin Steak with Portobello Mushrooms

Week 4

Days	Breakfast	Lunch	Snack	Dinner
29	Cinnamon Granola	Crisp Jicama and Red Lettuce Salad	Fresh Basil and Kalamata Hummus with Veggie Sticks	Hawaiian Meatballs
30	Hot Pepper and Salsa Frittata	Tomato Soup with Pasta and Chickpeas	Vanilla and Sweet Spice Dip with Dried Plums and Pecans	Tilapia with Lemon-Crumb Topping

The real wealth, and not gold and silver, is health.

Recipes

Breakfast

- Chocolate Pancakes
- Cinnamon Granola
- Hot Pepper and Salsa Frittata
- Peach and Raspberry Soufflé
- Slow-cooker fruity Oatmeal
- Apple Pie Spice Soufflé
- Berry-Infused French Toast Delight
- Protein-rich buckwheat Pancakes
- Blueberry-Banana Smoothie
- Blueberry-Banana Smoothie
- PB&J Smoothies
- Nutritious Oat-Nut Trail Bars

"When the diet is unhealthy, medicine is ineffective. When the diet is healthy, medicine becomes unnecessary."

Chocolate Pancakes

You can have these chocolate pancakes for breakfast or brunch. Serve them with warm syrup or honey whip.

- **Flour: 1½ cups**
- **Sugar: 1 cup**
- **Baking powder: 1 tsp**
- **Baking soda: ½ tsp**
- **Cocoa powder: ¼ cup**
- **Salt: ½ tsp**
- **Vegetable oil: ¼ cup**
- **Egg: 1**
- **Egg white: 1**
- **Buttermilk: ½ cup**
- **Vanilla: 1 tsp**
- **margarine: 2 tbsp**

Serves	6–8
cholesterol	34.68 mg
Calories	227.12
Sodium	177.18 mg
fat	11.05 grams
Saturated fat	3.23 grams
Dietary fibre	1.53 grams

Instructions

1. Take a medium bowl and mix flour, sugar, baking powder, baking soda, cocoa and salt in it. In another small bowl, whisk oil egg yolk buttermilk, and vanilla extract until smooth.

2. Pour the wet ingredients into the dry ones and stir with a beater or a whisk till the batter becomes even; let it stand for at least ten minutes.

3. Preheat a large griddle or frying pan over medium heat and grease it with margarine. Place ¼ cup of batter onto the heated surface. Cook until

the edges dry out and bubbles that burst appear on top then set for about three to five minutes in total after which flip the pancake and cook the other side an additional 1-2 minutes longer. serve immediately.

Cinnamon Granola

Granola made at home is not just an excellent breakfast choice but also a great snack. It can also be sprinkled on frozen yogurt or sherbet for a quick dessert.

- Rolled oats: 4 cups
- Oat bran: ¼ cup
- Flaxseed: ¼ cup
- Chopped walnuts: 1 cup
- Honey: ½ cup
- Brown sugar: ¼ cup
- Orange juice: 3 tbsp
- Canola oil: ¼ cup
- Salt: ¼ tsp
- Vanilla extract: 1 tbsp
- Ground cinnamon: 1 tbsp
- Dried cranberries: 1 cup
- Raisins: 1 cup

Serves	18
cholesterol	0.1 mg
Calories	347
Sodium	78.62 mg
fat	13 gram
Saturated fat	1.03 grams
Dietary fibre	8 grams

Instructions

1. Get your oven warmed up to 300 degrees Fahrenheit. Give a baking sheet with edges a gentle mist of cooking spray so nothing sticks.

2. Take a big mixing bowl and throw in your oats, oat bran, flaxseed, and walnuts, and mix. Then, in a little pot, heat the honey, brown sugar, orange juice, canola oil, and a pinch of salt on a low flame. Once it's warm, take it off the burner and mix in the vanilla.

3. . Drizzle that sweet, warm liquid all over your oat blend, giving it a good mix to make sure every bit is covered. Spread it all out nicely on your prepared baking sheet.

4. Let it bake for a good 45 minutes. Don't forget to stir it every 10 minutes so it cooks evenly. After it's done, jazz it up with a dash of cinnamon, and fold in the cranberries and raisins. Wait for it to cool down before you tuck it away in a container that seals tight.

Hot Pepper and Salsa Frittata

When you're looking for a shortcut, grab some low-sodium salsa from the health food or organic aisle at your local market, and prepare this.

- Olive oil: 2 tbsp
- Finely chopped red onion: ½ cup
- Minced jalapeño pepper: 1
- Egg substitute: ½ cup
- Egg whites: 4
- Skim milk: ¼ cup
- Grated Parmesan cheese: 3 tbsp
- Spicy salsa: ½ cup
- Chopped cilantro: 2 tbsp

Serves	3
cholesterol	7.6 mg
Calories	201.08
Sodium	29 1 mg
fat	12.47 grams
Saturated fat	2. 92 grams
Dietary fibre	1.53 grams

Instructions

1. Warm up some olive oil in a big nonstick frying pan on medium heat. Add onion jalapeno pepper: cook tender for about four minutes.

2. Beat egg substitute, egg whites, milk, and cheese together in a bowl. Pour this mixture into the skillet. Cook while moving a spatula around the edges of the pan until the eggs are softly set and the bottom is lightly browned.

3. Preheat broiler. Place under broiler for 4 to seven minutes or until top is browned; garnish with salsa and cilantro before serving right away.

Peach and Raspberry Soufflé

This lighter version of a soufflé is delicate and should be served immediately as it may fall quickly.

- **Chopped thawed frozen peaches: 1½ cups**
- **margarine: 2 tbsp**
- **Flour: 2 tbsp**
- **Salt: 1 tsp**
- **Sugar (divided): ¼ cup**
- **Raspberry jelly: 3 tbsp**
- **Egg yolk: 1**
- **Egg whites: 6**
- **Cream of tartar: ¼ tsp**

Serves	3
cholesterol	67.51 mg
Calories	292.91
Sodium	208.17 mg
fat	8.13 grams
Saturated fat	4.07 grams
Dietary fibre	2 grams

Instructions

1. Heat oven to 400°F; drain peaches reserving juice.

2. Start by warming up the saucepan on a medium flame and then gently melt the margarine in it. Stir in flour and salt; cook and stir for 3 minutes more. Add sugar one tablespoon at a time, reserved peach juice jelly: stir till thickened, remove from heat, and whisk in yolk plus peaches.

3. In a large bowl beat egg whites with salt cream of tartar till foamy Gradually add remaining sugar beating till stiff peaks form.

4. Fold small amounts of egg white into peach mixture then carefully fold in the rest of the egg whites Spray a two-quart casserole dish using non stick spray and pour batter into it Bake for thirty-five to forty-five minutes puffed up golden brown serve immediately.

Slow-cooker fruity Oatmeal

You can warm up leftover oatmeal in the microwave or use dried fruits like raisins or cranberries as an alternative

- Steel-cut oats: 2 cups
- Water: 4 cups
- Orange juice: 1½ cups
- Salt: ¼ tsp
- Ground cinnamon: ½ tsp
- Apples, peeled and chopped: 2
- Dried fruit bits: 1 cup
- Brown sugar: ½ cup
- Fat-free half-and-half: ½ cup

Serves	7
cholesterol	0.91 mg
Calories	358.31
Sodium	123.11 mg
fat	5.92 grams
Saturated fat	0.91 grams
Dietary fibre	7.39 grams

Instructions

1. The evening before serving, gently toast the oats in a small saucepan on low heat for approximately 5 to 8 minutes, ensuring to stir them often until they achieve a light golden hue. Transfer the toasted oats into a 2.5-quart slow cooker.

2. Incorporate all other ingredients, except the half-and-half and Cinnamon Granola, into the slow cooker. Mix thoroughly. Secure the lid and set the cooker to low, allowing the mixture to cook for a duration of 7 to 9 hours.

3. Upon waking, blend the half-and-half into the oat mixture and continue to cook for an additional 10 minutes. Garnish with Cinnamon Granola before serving.

Apple Pie Spice Soufflé

Enjoy the sweet scent of baking apple pie soufflé! Accompany with a glass of refreshing orange juice and some delicious chicken or turkey sausages for an ideal breakfast experience.

- **Applesauce: 1 cup**
- **Finely chopped apple: ½ cup**
- **Brown sugar: 2 tbsp**
- **Lemon juice: 2 tbsp**
- **Cinnamon: ½ tsp**
- **Nutmeg: ¼ tsp**
- **Cloves: ⅛ tsp**
- **Salt: ¼ tsp**
- **Egg yolk: 1**
- **Egg whites: 8**
- **Cream of tartar: ½ tsp**
- **Sugar: 3 tbsp**

Serves	4
cholesterol	55.42 mg
Calories	181.22
Sodium	270.82 mg
fat	1.29 grams
Saturated fat	0.41 grams
Dietary fibre	0.99 grams

Instructions

1. Preheat the oven to 400° F. Combine applesauce, chopped apple, brown sugar, lemon juice, cinnamon, nutmeg, cloves salt, and egg yolk in a medium bowl; mix well.

2. Beat egg whites with cream of tartar until foamy in a large separate bowl; gradually beat in sugar until stiff peaks form. Gently fold this mixture into the apple mixture.

3.. Spray the bottom of a 2-quart souffle dish with nonstick cooking spray then add the apple mixture inside it. Bake for 45-50 minutes or until soufflé is puffed up and golden brown. Serve immediately.

Berry-Infused French Toast Delight

- Thick slices of Honey-Wheat Sesame Bread
- Buttermilk: 1 cup
- Egg: 1
- Sugar (separated): 3 tbsp
- Part-skim ricotta cheese: ½ cup
- Frozen blueberries: ¼ cup
- Cinnamon: ½ tsp
- margarine: 2 tbsp

Serves	6
cholesterol	59.78 mg
Calories	272.41
Sodium	123.72 mg
fat	8.65 grams
Saturated fat	4 grams
Dietary fibre	2.91 grams

Instructions

1. Cut each bread slice from one side making sure not to go through all the way. Whisk buttermilk, egg, and one tablespoon of sugar together in a shallow dish.

2. Combine ricotta, cinnamon, and two tablespoons of sugar in a small bowl. Fold in the blueberries and stuff this mixture into the pocket of bread.

3. Start by warming up the saucepan on a medium flame and then gently melt the margarine in it. Dip this stuffed bread into the egg mixture ensuring it is well coated. Fry until golden brown and crispy, about 6-9

minutes, flipping once. Serve while hot.

Protein-rich buckwheat Pancakes

Buckwheat is a fruit seed that provides gluten-free flour rich in protein and fiber, which is good for cholesterol control.

- **Buttermilk: ½ cup**
- **Melted margarine: 2 tbsp**
- **Egg whites: 2**
- **Buckwheat flour: ½ cup**
- **All-purpose flour: ½ cup**
- **Baking powder: 1½ tsp**
- **Baking soda: ½ tsp**
- **Sugar: 3 tbsp**

Serves	4
cholesterol	17. 01 mg
Calories	215.88
Sodium	360.46 mg
fat	6.87 grams
Saturated fat	4 grams
Dietary fibre	1.93 grams

Instructions

1. Mix buttermilk, melted butter, and egg whites in a smaller bowl.

2. In another larger bowl combine flour, baking powder, baking soda, and sugar. Then add wet ingredients to the dry; stir just till moistened.

3. Heat sprayed skillet or griddle; pour ¼ cup portions of batter onto it. Cook until bubbles form and burst then turn and cook for another one to two minutes. Serve right away.

Blueberry-Banana Smoothie

- Skim milk: 1½ cups
- Banana: 1
- Blueberries: 1 cup
- Nonfat vanilla yogurt: 1 cup
- Ice cubes: 4

Serves	3
cholesterol	5.42 mg
Calories	273.42
Sodium	160 mg
fat	5 grams
Saturated fat	2.81 grams
Dietary fibre	3.74 grams

Instructions

1. Combine milk, banana, blueberries, and yogurt in a blender until smooth. Add ice and blend to thicken. Serve in glasses right away.

Apple-Cinnamon Smoothie

- Applesauce: 1 cup
- Vanilla yogurt: ½ cup
- Cinnamon: ½ tsp
- Peeled, chopped apple: 1
- Ice cubes: 4

Serves	2
cholesterol	3 mg
Calories	180
Sodium	46 mg
fat	1g
Saturated fat	0.45g
Dietary fibre	2.50g

Instructions

1. Combine applesauce, yogurt, cinnamon, and bite-sized apple pieces in a blender until smooth. Add ice as desired then blend again. serve.

PB&J Smoothies

Enjoy a cholesterol-free peanut butter smoothie, with low-fat options available.

- **Raspberry yogurt: 1 cup**
- **Skim milk: 1 cup**
- **Peanut butter: 3 tbsp**
- **Frozen vanilla yogurt: ½ cup**
- **Raspberry jelly: 2 tbsp**

Serves	2
cholesterol	4.3mg
Calories	167.2
Sodium	56 mg
fat	1.05 grams
Saturated fat	1.03 grams
Dietary fibre	3 grams

Instructions

1. Combine yogurt, milk, peanut butter, and frozen yogurt in blender until smooth. Mix in a jam just until marbled through it (the jelly). Fill glasses instantly and enjoy

Nutritious Oat-Nut Trail Bars

These snack bars are high-fiber wholesome treats that can also be used as on-the-go meals or taken to school lunches.

- **Brown sugar: 1 cup**
- **Canola oil: ¼ cup**
- **Egg: 1**
- **Orange juice: ½ cup**
- **Oatmeal: ¼ cup**
- **All-purpose flour: 1 cup**
- **Baking powder: 1 tsp**
- **Baking soda: 1 tsp**
- **Egg whites: 3**
- **Chopped walnuts: ½ cup**
- **Dried cranberries: ½ cup**
- **Golden raisins: ½ cup**

Yields	21 bars
cholesterol	9mg
Calories	123.21
Sodium	82mg
fat	3.54g
Saturated fat	0.27 g
Dietary fibre	2 g

Instructions

1. Preheat the oven to 300°f ; coat a baking dish (9″ x13″) with non-stick spray.
2. Mix brown sugar, oil, egg, and juice. Go ahead and toss in the oats, some flour, baking powder, and baking soda.
3. Whip the egg whites until it forms a peak then add to the mixture together with raisins and walnuts. Pour into the pan.
4. Bake for 45-55 minutes until set. Cool for 20 minutes; cut into bars and seal one by one.

Breads and Muffins

- Zucchini Nut Loaf
- Cinnamon Hazelnut Pastries
- Berry-Oat Coffee Cake
- Carrot-Oat Loaf
- Apple-Cranberry Nut Loaf
- Morning Delight Muffins
- Savory Cheddar and Herb Biscuits
- Hearty Whole-Grain Cornbread
- Oat-bran and Date Muffins
- Aromatic Pumpkin Bread

"There's no magic solution; you have to eat well and live a healthy lifestyle to be healthy and look healthy. That's all there is to it."

Zucchini Nut Loaf

In late summer, when you have more zucchini than you know what to do with, make a few loaves of this sweet bread. You can freeze them and enjoy them all winter long.

- **Canola oil: ¼ cup**
- **Sugar: ¼ cup**
- **Brown sugar: ½ cup**
- **Egg: 1**
- **Egg whites: 2**
- **Orange juice: ½ cup**
- **Vanilla: 2 tsp**
- **Grated zucchini: 1 cup**
- **Grated lemon zest: 1 tsp**
- **Wheat germ: 2 tbsp**
- **All-purpose flour: 1 cup**
- **Whole-wheat flour: 1 cup**
- **Baking powder: 1 tsp**
- **Baking soda: ½ tsp**
- **Salt: ½ tsp**
- **Cinnamon: 1 tsp**
- **Cloves: ¼ tsp**
- **Chopped walnuts: ½ cup**

Serves	12
cholesterol	18.01 mg
Calories	220.35
Sodium	127.63 mg
fat	9 grams
Saturated fat	0.70 grams
Dietary fibre	2.07 grams

Instructions

1. Preheat the oven to 350°F. Spray a 9″ × 5″ loaf pan with a flour-based nonstick spray; set aside.

2. In a large mixing bowl, whisk together the oil, sugars, egg, egg whites, orange juice, and vanilla until smooth. Stir in the grated zucchini, lemon zest, and wheat germ.

3. Sift together the all-purpose flour, whole-wheat flour, baking powder,

baking soda, salt, cinnamon and cloves. Add these dry ingredients to the wet mixture and stir just until combined; fold in chopped walnuts. Pour batter into the prepared pan.

4. Bake for 55–65 minutes or until golden brown and the toothpick inserted in comes out clean from the center of the loaf. After baking remove the loaf from the pan; let cool on a wire rack.

Cinnamon Hazelnut Pastries

Scones are essentially sweet biscuits–and you can add your choice of dried fruits or nuts.

- **All-purpose flour: 1 cup**
- **Whole-wheat flour: 1 cup**
- **Brown sugar: 1 cup**
- **Cinnamon: 1 tsp**
- **Baking powder: 1 tsp**
- **Baking soda: ½ tsp**
- **plant sterol margarine: 3 tbsp**
- **Canola oil: 3 tbsp**
- **Egg: 1**
- **Buttermilk: ½ cup**
- **Vanilla: 1 tsp**
- **Dried cranberries: ½ cup**
- **Chopped hazelnuts: ½ cup**
- **Milk: 1 tbsp**

Serves	8
cholesterol	39.01 mg
Calories	285.02
Sodium	192.16 mg
fat	15 grams
Saturated fat	3.98 grams
Dietary fibre	3 grams

Instructions

1. Preheat your oven to 400°F; line a cookie sheet with parchment paper.

2. In a large mixing bowl combine flour with brown sugar, cinnamon, baking powder, and baking soda. Incorporate the margarine until the mixture achieves a fine crumb texture.

3. In another small bowl beat oil, eggs, buttermilk, and vanilla. Add this mixture to dry ingredients, stirring just until moistened.

4. Stir in cranberries and hazelnuts gently. On a floured surface knead dough lightly. Shape into an 8-inch circle on a cookie sheet. Cut into wedges spacing slightly apart. Brush tops with milk. Bake for 15-18 minutes until golden brown. Cool for five minutes before serving.

Berry-Oat Coffee Cake

This coffee cake is loaded with fruit, oats, and nuts–making it a delightful treat, especially when served warm.

- **Brown sugar: ½ cup**
- **Cinnamon: 1½ tsp**
- **Oatmeal: 1 cup**
- **Chopped walnuts: ½ cup**
- **Canola oil (divided): 6 tbsp**
- **plant sterol margarine: 2 tbsp**
- **Blueberries: 1 cup**
- **Dried cranberries: ½ cup**
- **Egg: 1**
- **Egg whites: 2**
- **Buttermilk: ¼ cup**
- **Orange juice: ¼ cup**
- **Sugar: ½ cup**
- **All-purpose flour: 1 cup**
- **Whole-wheat flour: 1 cup**
- **Baking powder: 2 tsp**
- **Baking soda: 1 tsp**

Serves	14
cholesterol	18.09 mg
Calories	262.87
Sodium	153.22 mg
fat	11.34 grams
Saturated fat	2 grams
Dietary fibre	3.02 grams

Instructions

1. Preheat your oven to 350°F. Spray the bottom only of a 13″ × 9″ baking pan with flour-based nonstick spray; set aside.

2. In a medium bowl, mix brown sugar, cinnamon, oatmeal, and walnuts. Melt canola oil and margarine together in a small saucepan; pour over the oat mixture, stirring until crumbs form. Stir in blueberries and cranberries; set aside.

3. In a large bowl, combine remaining oil, eggs, buttermilk, orange juice, and sugar; beat well. Add flour, baking powder, and baking soda; stir just until moistened by dry ingredients.

4. Spread batter into prepared pan. Even sprinkle the oatmeal mixture on top. Bake for 30-40 minutes or until the cake is golden brown and the toothpick comes out clean when inserted into it. Serve warm.

Carrot-Oat Loaf

This loaf has all the flavors of carrot cake but with less sweetness–it's perfect for a chicken salad sandwich.

- **Finely chopped carrots: 1½ cups**
- **Water: 1 cup**
- **All-purpose flour: 1½ cups**
- **Oatmeal: ¼ cup**
- **Oat bran: 2 tbsp**
- **Brown sugar: ½ cup**
- **Sugar: ⅓ cup**
- **Salt: ½ tsp**
- **Baking powder: 1 tsp**
- **Baking soda: ½ tsp**
- **Cinnamon: ½ tsp**
- **Ginger: ½ tsp**
- **Applesauce: ½ cup**
- **Canola oil: ¼ cup**
- **Egg whites: 2**
- **Chopped walnuts: ½ cup**

Serves	13
cholesterol	0.0 mg
Calories	245.03
Sodium	109.07 mg
fat	9 grams
Saturated fat	0.42 grams
Dietary fibre	2.04 grams

Instructions

1. Begin by preheating your oven to a temperature of 350 degrees Fahrenheit. Ready a loaf pan measuring 9 by 5 inches by spraying it with a nonstick coating that contains flour.

2. Place the carrots in a small saucepan, pour in some water, and bring to a boil. Cook until they are soft, which should take approximately 5 to 7 minutes. After draining,

puree the carrots until they achieve a smooth consistency, then set aside.

3. Take a sizable mixing bowl and combine the following dry ingredients: flour, oatmeal, oat bran, both types of sugar, salt, baking powder, baking soda, cinnamon, and ginger. In a separate bowl, amalgamate the pureed carrots, applesauce, oil, and egg whites. Stir this wet mixture into the dry ingredients until they are barely combined, then gently incorporate the walnuts.

4. Transfer the prepared batter into the loaf pan and bake it for a duration of 55 to 65 minutes, or until the loaf attains a rich golden hue. If you poke the middle with a toothpick and it emerges without any gooey bits, you're good to go! Once baked, remove the loaf from the pan and let it cool on a wire rack.

Apple-Cranberry Nut Loaf

This is a flavorful loaf that makes use of autumn apples and is quick to serve for breakfast.

- **Apples, peeled and diced: 2**
- **Sugar: ¼ cup**
- **Brown sugar: ½ cup**
- **Canola oil: ¼ cup**
- **Egg: 1**
- **Vanilla: 2 tsp**
- **Apple juice, divided: 1 cup**
- **All-purpose flour: 1¼ cups**
- **Whole-wheat flour: ¼ cup**
- **Baking powder: 1 tsp**
- **Baking soda: ½ tsp**
- **Cinnamon: 1 tsp**
- **Dried cranberries: ½ cup**
- **Fresh chopped cranberries: ½ cup**
- **Chopped walnuts: ½ cup**
- **Powdered sugar: 1 cup**

Serves	12
cholesterol	18.73 mg
Calories	266.72
Sodium	89.75 mg
fat	9 grams
Saturated fat	0.68 grams
Dietary fibre	2.71 grams

Instructions

1. Preheat your oven to 350°F. Prepare a 9" × 5" loaf pan by greasing it with a nonstick spray which contains flour.

2. In a sizable mixing bowl, blend together the apples with a quarter cup of sugar. Allow the mixture to rest for a quarter of an hour. Proceed to incorporate the brown sugar, oil, egg, vanilla extract, and a cup of apple juice, ensuring thorough mixing.

3. In another bowl; mix together flour, baking powder, baking soda, cinnamon, cranberries, and walnuts. Fold this into the apple mixture until just combined.

4. Then transfer the batter into the prepared loaf pan and bake for approximately fifty-five to sixty-five minutes or until it turns golden-brown outside and inside when tested with a toothpick comes out clean. Remove from the pan and cool on a wire rack.

5. In another smaller bowl blend powdered sugar with the remaining quarter cup apple juice and drizzle over warm loaf. Allow cooling before serving.

Morning Delight Muffins

Relish the soft texture of these nutritious muffins, packed with fiber and vital nutrients. Best served warm with a touch of creamy honey. Simply irresistible!

- **Plain flour: 1 cup**
- **Whole-wheat flour: 1 cup**
- **Oat bran: 2 tbsp**
- **Ground flaxseed: 2 tbsp**
- **Granulated sugar: ½ cup**
- **Brown sugar: ½ cup**
- **Cinnamon: 2 tsp**
- **Nutmeg: ¼ tsp**
- **Baking powder: 1½ tsp**
- **Baking soda: 1 tsp**
- **Peeled, chopped apples: 2**
- **Shredded carrots: 1 cup**
- **Applesauce: ½ cup**
- **Egg: 1**
- **Egg white: 1**
- **Low-fat sour cream: ¼ cup**
- **Canola oil: ¼ cup**
- **Vanilla extract: 2 tsp**
- **Dried cranberries: 1 cup**
- **Chopped walnuts: 1 cup**

Serves	20
cholesterol	14.12 mg
Calories	212.2
Sodium	121.09mg
fat	9 g
Saturated fat	0.92g
Dietary fibre	2.78g

Instructions

1. Set your oven's temperature to 375°F. Line 18 muffin cups with liners and keep them ready. In a large mixing bowl, whisk together the variety of flours, oat bran, milled flaxseed, both kinds of sugar, cinnamon, nutmeg, baking powder, and baking soda until well-blended.

2. In another bowl, combine the apples, carrots, applesauce, whole egg, egg white,

Sour cream, canola oil, and vanilla extract until the mixture is homogeneous. Mix this with the flour mixture, stirring just until the dry ingredients are moistened. Gently mix the cranberries and walnuts into the batter.

3. Pour the batter into the prepared muffin cups, filling each to 1/4 full. Bake for 15–25 minutes, or until the muffins are golden brown and a toothpick inserted in the center comes out clean. Shift the muffins over to a cooling grid and let them chill out for a bit.

Savory Cheddar and Herb Biscuits

Experience the pleasure of these freshly baked biscuits. Complement them with a herbal nonfat cream cheese for an enhanced taste.

- Plain flour: 1½ cups
- Whole-wheat flour: ½ cup
- Baking powder: 1½ tsp
- Baking soda: ½ tsp
- Garlic salt: ¼ tsp
- Canola oil: ¼ cup
- Egg white: 1
- Buttermilk: ¾ cup
- Grated low-fat extra-sharp Cheddar cheese: 1 cup
- Chopped fresh rosemary: 1 tbsp
- Fresh thyme leaves: 1 tbsp
- plant sterol margarine: 1 tbsp
- Chopped flat-leaf parsley: 1 tbsp

Serves	Yields 8 biscuits
cholesterol	8.1 mg
Calories	220.31
Sodium	282.13mg
fat	9.76 g
Saturated fat	2.92g
Dietary fibre	1.69 g

Instructions

1. Preheat your oven to 400°F. Arrange parchment paper on a baking tray and set aside.

2. In a sizable bowl, mix the flour, baking powder, baking soda, and garlic salt. In a smaller bowl, whisk together the oil, egg white, and buttermilk. Add the wet ingredients to the dry ones, stirring until just moist.

3. Incorporate the Cheddar cheese, rosemary, and thyme into the mixture. Drop the dough in eight portions onto the baking tray. Pop it in the oven for about 15 to 20 minutes, or just until it's nicely toasted to a light golden hue.

4. Melt margarine in a microwave-safe container, mix in the parsley, and brush over the hot biscuits. Allow the biscuits to cool on a rack for a few minutes before serving.

Hearty Whole-Grain Cornbread

Freshly baked, this cornbread is an excellent accompaniment to whipped honey or a dollop of zesty salsa.

- Plain flour: ¼ cup
- Whole-wheat flour: ½ cup
- Brown sugar: ¼ cup
- Baking powder: 2 tsp
- Baking soda: 1 tsp
- Cornmeal: 1 cup
- Oat bran: ¼ cup
- Egg: 1
- Egg whites: 2
- Honey: ¼ cup
- Buttermilk: 1 cup
- Canola oil: ¼ cup

Serves	10
cholesterol	23.99mg
Calories	259.77
Sodium	272.96mg
fat	8.2 g
Saturated fat	0.98 g
Dietary fibre	3.2 g

Instructions

1. Heat the oven to 400°F. Coat a 9-inch square baking pan with some non stick spray before you start. In a large bowl, combine the flour, brown sugar, baking powder, baking soda, cornmeal, and oat bran.

2. In a smaller bowl, beat the egg, egg whites, honey, buttermilk, and oil. Gently stir this liquid mixture into the dry ingredients until just blended.

3. Pour the batter into the prepared dish, smoothing the top. Pop it in the oven and let it cook for about 25 to 35 minutes. You'll know it's done

when it's got that perfect golden-brown color.

Oat-bran and Date Muffins

Enjoy the natural sweetness and soluble fiber of dates in these wholesome muffins, perfect for a nutritious treat.

- Plain flour: 1¼ cups
- Rolled oats: ½ cup
- Oat bran: ¼ cup
- Baking powder: 1½ tsp
- Baking soda: 1 tsp
- Brown sugar: ¾ cup
- Egg: 1
- Canola oil: ¼ cup
- Applesauce: ¾ cup
- Grated orange zest: 1 tsp
- Finely chopped dates: 1 cup
- Chopped hazelnuts: ½ cup

Serves	14 muffins
cholesterol	18.56 mg
Calories	233.31
Sodium	162.36mg
fat	8.76g
Saturated fat	0.80g
Dietary fibre	4.27g

Instructions

1. Heat the oven to 350°F. Get your 12-cup muffin tray ready by popping in some paper cups. In a large bowl, combine the flour, oats, oat bran, baking powder, baking soda, and brown sugar.

2. In another bowl, whisk the egg, oil, applesauce, and orange zest. Add to the dry ingredients, stirring until just moist. Fold in the dates and hazelnuts.

3. Spoon the batter into the muffin cups, filling them to the top. Bake for 25–35 minutes, until firm to the touch and a toothpick inserted comes out clean. Allow the muffins to cool on wire racks after removal from the pan.

Aromatic Pumpkin Bread

Infuse your home with the delightful scent of baking pumpkin bread, with an equally captivating taste.

- **Brown sugar: ½ cup**
- **Sugar: ¼ cup**
- **Canola oil: ¼ cup**
- **Egg: 1**
- **Egg whites: 2**
- **Vanilla extract: 2 tsp**
- **Canned solid-pack no-salt pumpkin: 1 cup**
- **Plain flour: 1¼ cups**
- **Whole-wheat flour: ½ cup**
- **Baking powder: 1 tsp**
- **Baking soda: ½ tsp**
- **Cinnamon, divided: 1 tsp**
- **Nutmeg: ¼ tsp**
- **Cardamom: ¼ tsp**
- **Sugar: 2 tbsp**

Serves	14
cholesterol	34.12 mg
Calories	168.01
Sodium	111.66 mg
fat	4.56 g
Saturated fat	0.73 g
Dietary fibre	1.21 g

Instructions

1. Warm the oven to 350°F. Coat a 9" × 5" loaf pan with nonstick spray.

2. In a large bowl, cream the brown sugar, ¼ cup sugar, oil, egg, egg whites, and vanilla. Stir in the pumpkin for a smooth mixture.

3. Sift together the flour, baking powder, baking soda, ½ teaspoon cinnamon, nutmeg, and cardamom. Gradually add these dry ingredients to the pumpkin mixture, beating until smooth.

4. Transfer the batter to the pan. Mix 2 tablespoons sugar with ½ teaspoon cinnamon and sprinkle on top. Place in the oven and allow to cook for an hour to an hour and ten minutes, ensuring it's ready when a toothpick inserted into the center emerges without any residue. Let the bread rest on a wire rack to cool prior to cutting it into slices.

Poultry

- **Chicken Breasts with Salsa**
- **Asian Chicken Stir-Fry**
- **Mashed Bean-Topped Chicken Breasts**
- **New Potatoes with Chicken Breasts**
- **Tomato Sauce Poached Chicken**
- **Hazelnut-Crusted Chicken Breasts**
- **Turkey Stuffed with Prune**
- **Texas BBQ Chicken Thighs**
- **Turkey Cutlets Florentine**
- **Turkey Cutlets Parmesan**
- **Chicken Pesto with Hazelnuts**
- **Chilled Chicken with Cherry Tomato Sauce**

"Maintaining good health is a responsibility; otherwise, we won't be able to keep our mind clear."

Chicken Breasts with Salsa

Whole-grain cereal is an excellent source of folic acid, which helps lower homocysteine levels. It also makes a great crunchy coating for chicken breasts.

- **Lime juice, divided: 2 tablespoons**
- **Egg white: 1**
- **Whole-grain cereal, crushed: 1 cup**
- **Dried thyme leaves: 1 teaspoon**
- **Pepper: ¼ teaspoon**
- **Four boneless, skinless chicken breasts, each weighing 4 ounces.**
- **Super Spicy Salsa: 1 cup**
- **Jalapeño pepper, minced: 1**

Serves	4
cholesterol	87.3 mg
Calories	269.07
Sodium	136.65 mg
fat	4.51 grams
Saturated fat	2 grams
Dietary fibre	4.83 grams

Instructions

1. Preheat your oven to 375°F. Prepare a cookie sheet with a wire rack and set it aside. In a small bowl, mix 1 tablespoon of lime juice with the egg white and beat until frothy. On a shallow plate, combine the crushed cereal, thyme, and pepper.

2. Dip the chicken breasts into the egg white mixture, then coat them with the cereal mixture. Position the prepared chicken, which has been coated, onto the ready baking tray. Bake for 20–25 minutes, or until the chicken is

fully cooked and the coating is crisp.

3. Meanwhile, in a small saucepan, combine the remaining 1 tablespoon of lime juice, salsa, and minced jalapeño pepper. Heat the mixture, stirring occasionally, until warmed through. Serve the salsa mixture over the baked chicken.

Asian Chicken Stir-Fry

Yellow summer squash, similar to zucchini, has a tender skin and a mild, sweet flavor.

- **Boneless, skinless chicken breasts: 2 (5-ounce each)**
- **Low-Sodium Chicken Broth: ½ cup**
- **Low-sodium soy sauce: 1 tablespoon**
- **Cornstarch: 1 tablespoon**
- **Sherry: 1 tablespoon**
- **Peanut oil: 2 tablespoons**
- **Onion, sliced: 1**
- **Garlic cloves, minced: 3**
- **Ginger root, grated: 1 tablespoon**
- **Snow peas: 1 cup**
- **Canned sliced water chestnuts, drained: ½ cup**
- **Yellow summer squash, sliced: 1**
- **Chopped unsalted peanuts: ¼ cup**

Serves	5
cholesterol	39. 34 mg
Calories	253.48
Sodium	201.06 mg
fat	13 grams
Saturated fat	2.11 grams
Dietary fibre	4 grams

Instructions

1. Cut the chicken into thin pieces and place them to the side. In a small bowl, combine the chicken broth, soy sauce, cornstarch, and sherry; set aside.

2. In a large skillet or wok, heat the peanut oil over medium-high heat. Add the chicken and stir-fry until almost cooked, about 3–4 minutes, then remove to a plate. Add the onion, garlic, and ginger root to the skillet and stir-fry for another 4 minutes. Then, add the snow peas, water chestnuts,

and squash; stir-fry for an additional 2 minutes.

3. Stir the chicken broth mixture and add it to the skillet along with the chicken. Stir-fry for another 3–4 minutes, or until the chicken is fully cooked and the sauce has thickened and become bubbly. Sprinkle with chopped peanuts and serve immediately.

Mashed Bean-Topped Chicken Breasts

To delight your guests visually, arrange the bean puree on each dish and crown it with a perfectly sautéed chicken breast.

- **Olive oil, divided: 3 tablespoons**
- **Onion, chopped: 1**
- **Garlic cloves, minced: 3**
- **One can (14 ounces) of cannellini beans with reduced sodium content, thoroughly drained and rinsed.**
- **Flat-leaf parsley, chopped: ½ cup**
- **Dried oregano leaves: ½ teaspoon**
- **Dried basil leaves: 1 teaspoon**
- **Grated Parmesan cheese: ¼ cup**
- **Flour: 3 tablespoons**
- **White pepper: ¼ teaspoon**
- **Boneless, skinless chicken breasts: 6 (4-ounce each)**

Serves	6
cholesterol	89.34 mg
Calories	316.30
Sodium	144.62 mg
fat	11.61 grams
Saturated fat	2.72 grams
Dietary fibre	3.01 grams

Instructions

1. Start by warming a tablespoon of olive oil in a medium saucepan, then toss in chopped onion and minced garlic, sautéing until soft, which should take about 5 minutes. After draining the cannellini beans, give them a good rinse and drain once more.

2. Pop the beans into the saucepan along with a mix of parsley, oregano, and basil, stirring until everything's piping hot, around 5 minutes. Crush the

beans with a potato masher until nicely mashed, then dial the heat down to a low simmer.

3. On a flat plate, blend together Parmesan cheese, flour, and a dash of white pepper. Coat each chicken breast in this cheesy blend. In a large skillet, heat the remaining olive oil over a medium flame.

4. Lay the chicken in the skillet, letting it cook undisturbed for 5 minutes. Gently flip the chicken and allow it to cook for another 4–6 minutes until it's cooked all the way through. Serve atop the warm bean mash.

New Potatoes with Chicken Breasts

This simple one-pan dish is a symphony of flavors, with mustard bringing a zesty kick to tender chicken and crispy potatoes.

- Small new red potatoes: 12
- Olive oil: 2 tablespoons
- White pepper: 1 teaspoon
- Garlic cloves, minced: 4
- Dried oregano leaves: 1 teaspoon
- Dijon mustard: 2 tablespoons
- Four boneless, skinless chicken breasts, each weighing 4 ounces.
- Cherry tomatoes: 1 cup

Serves	6
cholesterol	63.45 mg
Calories	399.93
Sodium	148 mg
fat	10 grams
Saturated fat	2.3 grams
Dietary fibre	5.37 grams

Instructions

1. Heat your oven to 400°F and line a roasting pan with parchment. Give the new potatoes a good scrub and slice them in half, arranging them in the pan.

2. Whisk together olive oil, white pepper, minced garlic, oregano, and Dijon mustard in a small bowl. Pour half this mixture over the potatoes, tossing to coat them well. Roast for 20 minutes.

3. Cut the chicken breasts into quarters and, after the potatoes have had their time, add the chicken to the pan, mixing it with the potatoes. Pour the

remaining oil blend over the surface. Return it to the oven for an additional 15 minutes.

4. Toss in some cherry tomatoes and roast for an additional 5–10 minutes until the potatoes are tender and browned, and the chicken is fully cooked.

Tomato Sauce Poached Chicken

Tarragon, with its unique mild licorice flavor, is a fantastic complement to chicken and tomatoes, creating a delightful dish.

- **Brown rice: 1 cup**
- **Water: 2 cups**
- **Olive oil: 2 tablespoons**
- **Onion, chopped: 1**
- **Garlic cloves, minced: 3**
- **Plum tomatoes, chopped: 2 cups**
- **Dried tarragon: ½ teaspoon**
- **Dry red wine: ¼ cup**
- **No-salt tomato paste: 3 tablespoons**
- **Low-Sodium Chicken Broth: 1 cup**
- **Salt: ¼ teaspoon**
- **Pepper: ¼ teaspoon**
- **Boneless, skinless chicken thighs, sliced: 3 (5-ounce each)**

Serves	4
cholesterol	62.72 mg
Calories	273.33
Sodium	130 mg
fat	9.61 grams
Saturated fat	1.74 grams
Dietary fibre	2.72 grams

Instructions

1. In a medium saucepan, mix rice and water and bring it to a boil. Once boiling, reduce the heat to a simmer, cover, and let it cook for 30–40 minutes until the rice is tender.

2. While the rice cooks, warm some olive oil in a large saucepan over medium heat. Add chopped onion and minced garlic, cooking until they're just tender. Stir in chopped plum tomatoes, dried tarragon, a splash of dry red wine, no-salt tomato paste, chicken broth, and a pinch of salt and

pepper. Maintain a gentle simmer, occasionally stirring the mixture.

3. Add sliced chicken thighs to the sauce and let it come back to a gentle simmer. Cover the pan, reduce the heat, and let the chicken poach for 15–20 minutes until it's completely cooked.

4. Serve the poached chicken over the fluffy rice. If you have leftover tomato paste, freeze it in tablespoon-sized portions for up to 3 months.

Hazelnut-Crusted Chicken Breasts

For a quick dinner that's sure to impress, try this super-fast dish. Pair it with a fresh spinach salad and some crunchy breadsticks for a complete meal.

- **Boneless, skinless chicken breasts: 2 (4-ounce each)**
- **Salt: Pinch**
- **Pepper: Pinch**
- **Dijon mustard: 1 tablespoon**
- **Egg white: 1**
- **Chopped hazelnuts: ¼ cup**
- **Olive oil: 1 tablespoon**

Serves	2
cholesterol	67.78 mg
Calories	281. 67
Sodium	265.30 mg
fat	17.11 grams
Saturated fat	1.88 grams
Dietary fibre	1.51 grams

Instructions

1. Place the chicken between wax paper and pound it to a ¼-inch thickness. Season the flattened chicken with salt and pepper, then spread a bit of mustard on each side.

2. Whisk an egg white until it's foamy in a small bowl. Dip the chicken into the egg white, then coat it with hazelnuts, making sure both sides are well-covered.

3. Warm a bit of olive oil in a frying pan on a moderate flame. Cook the chicken for 3 minutes without moving it, then carefully flip it over and

cook for another 1–3 minutes until it's fully cooked and the nuts are toasted. Serve it up right away!

> **Healthy Hints**
>
> - Dijon mustard is a robust condiment, quite different from the yellow mustard used on hot dogs, and it's packed with nutrients like potassium, calcium, and niacin while being low in fat and cholesterol.

Turkey Stuffed with Prune

Packed with pectin, prunes surpass even oat bran in their ability to soak up cholesterol in the intestines.

- **Olive oil: 3 tbsp**
- **Onion, chopped: 1**
- **Garlic cloves, minced: 3**
- **Finely chopped pitted prunes: 1 cup**
- **Salt: ½ tsp**
- **Pepper: ½ tsp**
- **Chopped hazelnuts: ½ cup**
- **Turkey cutlets: 6 (3-ounce each)**
- **Flour: 2 tbsp**
- **Low-Sodium Chicken Broth: ½ cup**
- **Dry white wine: ¼ cup**
- **Dried thyme leaves: ½ tsp**
- **Lemon juice: 1 tbsp**

Serves	6
cholesterol	60. 81 mg
Calories	330.80
Sodium	93. 54 mg
fat	15. 56 grams
Saturated fat	2.10 grams
Dietary fibre	1.43 grams

Instructions

1. Begin by warming a tablespoon of olive oil in a small pot over a medium flame. Toss in chopped onion and minced garlic, sautéing until they're just tender, which should take around 4 minutes. Introduce the prunes to the mix, seasoning with a pinch of salt and pepper. Let them cook until they start to swell, about 3 to 4 minutes, then toss in the chopped nuts and take the pan off the heat. Give it about 20 minutes to cool down.

2. Next, lay out the turkey cutlets flat and distribute the pruned mixture evenly across them. Roll them up snugly, securing them with twine or toothpicks. Lightly coat the rolls in flour.

3. Heat the remaining olive oil in a bigger skillet, browning the turkey rolls evenly for around 4 to 5 minutes. Then pour in the broth, wine, and thyme. Cover up and let it braise for 6 to 8 minutes until the turkey is tender and cooked through. Finally, splash in some lemon juice and serve it up hot.

Texas BBQ Chicken Thighs

- Olive oil: 2 tbsp
- Onion, chopped: 1
- Garlic cloves, minced: 4
- Jalapeño pepper, minced: 1
- Orange juice: ¼ cup
- Low-sodium soy sauce: 1 tbsp
- Apple cider vinegar: 2 tbsp
- Brown sugar: 2 tbsp
- Dijon mustard: 2 tbsp
- Crushed tomatoes (14-ounce can), undrained: 1 can
- Cumin: ½ tsp
- Chili powder: 1 tbsp
- Pepper: ¼ tsp
- Boneless, skinless chicken thighs: 6 (4-ounce each)
- Cornstarch: 3 tbsp
- Water: ¼ cup

Serves	6
cholesterol	97.33 mg
Calories	238.64 mg
Sodium	280.31 mg
fat	9.73 grams
Saturated fat	2.01 grams
Dietary fibre	2.01 grams

Instructions

1. Warm up a bit of olive oil in a skillet over medium heat. Cook the chopped onion and minced garlic until they're just right, about 4 minutes, then transfer them to a 3–4 quart slow cooker. Add the fiery jalapeño, orange zest, soy sauce, vinegar, brown sugar, mustard, tomatoes, and a blend of cumin, chili powder, and pepper.

2. Nestle the chicken thighs in the sauce, making sure they're completely submerged. Seal the lid and let it cook on low for 8–10 hours, until the chicken is perfectly done.

3. To thicken the sauce, mix cornstarch with water until smooth, then stir it into the slow cooker. Crank the heat up to high and let it bubble for another 15–20 minutes. serve.

Some individuals might regard chicken thighs as overly rich in fat. However, it's worth noting that these cuts have a relatively modest fat content, with only 11 grams per 4 ounces, which is lower than the fat content in an equivalent serving of beef, lamb, or pork.

Turkey Cutlets Florentine

Florentine-style means you're in for a spinach treat, loaded with antioxidants and fiber, and oh-so-tasty!

- Egg white, beaten: 1
- Dry breadcrumbs: ½ cup
- White pepper: 1 tsp
- Grated Parmesan cheese: 2 tbsp
- Turkey cutlets: 6 (4 ounces each)
- Olive oil: 2 tbsp
- Garlic cloves, minced: 2
- Fresh baby spinach (8-ounce bags): 2 bags
- Ground nutmeg: 1 tsp
- Shredded Jarlsberg cheese: 1 cup

Serves	6
cholesterol	85.21 mg
Calories	249.57
Sodium	236.98
fat	9.52 grams
Saturated fat	2. 30 grams
Dietary fibre	2.13 grams

Instructions

1. Whip up some egg whites in a bowl until it's frothy. Mix breadcrumbs, a dash of pepper, and Parmesan on a plate.

2. If your turkey cutlets are on the thick side, place them between wax paper and gently pound them thinner. Dip each cutlet first into the egg white, then coat with the breadcrumb mix.

3. In a large pan, heat olive oil over a medium-high flame. Cook the

turkey for 4 minutes, flip it, and give it another 4–6 minutes. Move the cutlets to a plate and tent with foil to keep them warm.

4. Toss the garlic into the pan and cook for a minute. Add spinach and a pinch of nutmeg, stirring until the spinach wilts, which takes about 4–5 minutes. Sprinkle Jarlsberg cheese over the top, cover with the turkey, and remove from heat. Let it stand for a couple of minutes to let the cheese melt, then it's ready to serve.

> **Healthy Hints**
>
> - opt for smaller amounts of strongly flavored cheeses, like extra-sharp Cheddar, Gruyère, or Cotija, and consider grating or shredding to maximize taste while minimizing quantity.

Turkey Cutlets Parmesan

- **Egg white: 1**
- **Dry breadcrumbs: ¼ cup**
- **Pepper: 1 tsp**
- **Grated Parmesan cheese: 4 tbsp (divided)**
- **Turkey cutlets: 6 (4 ounces each)**
- **Olive oil: 2 tbsp**
- **No salt tomato sauce (15-ounce can): 1 can**
- **Dried Italian seasoning: 1 tsp**
- **Finely shredded part-skim mozzarella cheese: ½ cup**

Serves	2
cholesterol	90.13 mg
Calories	285.42
Sodium	218.90 mg
fat	11 grams
Saturated fat	3.70 grams
Dietary fibre	2 grams

Instructions

1. 1. Preheat your oven to 350°F and prepare a 2-quart baking dish with a spritz of nonstick spray.

2. Beat an egg white until it's nice and frothy. Combine breadcrumbs, a hint of pepper, and some Parmesan on a plate. Coat the turkey cutlets with egg white, then breadcrumb and mix.

3. In a sizable pan, warm up some olive oil in a medium setting. Toss in the turkey slices and give them a good sear on each side, letting them

cook for roughly 2 to 3 minutes. After they've got a nice color, transfer them to the baking dish you've got ready. Next, pour the tomato sauce into the pan and sprinkle some Italian herbs in there. Heat it up until it starts bubbling away.

4. Drizzle the cutlets in the baking dish with the sauce, and sprinkle the mozzarella and the rest of the Parmesan on top. Pop it in the oven for about 25 to 35 minutes, or wait until you see the sauce bubbling and the cheese getting all melty and starting to get that golden-brown look. you can totally have it with some pasta on the side.

Chicken Pesto with Hazelnuts

Hazelnuts not only lower LDL cholesterol but also add a delightful flavor to pesto sauce.

- Fresh basil leaves, packed: 1 cup
- Toasted chopped hazelnuts: ¼ cup
- Garlic cloves, chopped: 2
- Olive oil: 2 tbsp
- Water: 1 tbsp
- Grated Parmesan cheese: ¼ cup
- LowSodium Chicken Broth: ½ cup
- Boneless, skinless chicken breasts: 12 ounces
- Angel hair pasta (12-ounce package): 1 package

Serves	6
cholesterol	39.99 mg
Calories	377.69
Sodium	109 mg
fat	11. 12 grams
Saturated fat	2.01 grams
Dietary fibre	2.43 grams

Instructions

1. Begin by heating a pot of water seasoned with salt to a boil. In a blender or processor, blitz basil, hazelnuts, and garlic until finely chopped. Add in olive oil and water to form a paste, then mix in Parmesan cheese.

2. Simmer chicken broth in a skillet. Slice chicken into strips and simmer in the broth. Meanwhile, toss the pasta into the boiling water and cook

until al dente. Drain and combine with the chicken, cooking for a more. Stir in the basil mixture, take it off the heat, and mix until saucy.

Chilled Chicken with Cherry Tomato Sauce

This makes for an ideal dish on a warm summer day. Begin by preparing the chicken in advance, and when it's time to serve, promptly whip up the sauce.

- Fresh thyme leaves: 2 tsp
- LowSodium Chicken Broth: ½ cup
- Boneless, skinless chicken breasts: 12 ounces
- Olive oil: 1 tbsp
- Garlic cloves, minced: 3
- Cherry tomatoes: 2 cups
- Nosalt tomato juice: ½ cup
- Fresh basil, chopped: ½ cup
- Low-fat sour cream: ¼ cup
- White pepper: ½ tsp

Serves	3
cholesterol	77. 76 mg
Calories	Serves 6–8
Sodium	219.59
fat	9.67 grams
Saturated fat	3 grams
Dietary fibre	1.99 grams

Instructions

1. 1. Simmer thyme and chicken broth in a large pan. Poach the chicken until done, then transfer it to a dish, cover it with the liquid, and chill for at least 8 hours.

2. When it's time to eat, sauté garlic in olive oil for a minute. Add cherry tomatoes and cook until they burst. Mix in tomato juice, basil, sour cream, and pepper.

3. Slice the chilled chicken, arrange it on a plate, and top with the warm tomato sauce.

Salads

- **Charred Petite Beet Medley Salad**
- **Crisp Jicama and Red Lettuce Salad**
- **Warm New Potato Salad**
- **Hearty Wheat Berry Salad**
- **Pasta Salad with Crisp Vegetables**
- **French-Style Lentil Rice Salad**
- **Low-Fat Red Bean Salad with Taco Chips**
- **Crab and Edamame Salad with Surimi**
- **Apple Coleslaw**
- **Citrus Salad**
- **Black-Eyed Pea Salad**

"Health is the first wealth."

Charred Petite Beet Medley Salad

This delightful salad showcases the vibrant red hue of charred beets set against a backdrop of creamy white yogurt and crisp green romaine leaves, finished with a sprinkle of toasted walnuts for garnish.

- Baby beets: 8
- Olive oil: 2 tbsp
- White wine vinegar: 2 tbsp
- Salt: ¼ tsp
- White pepper: ¼ tsp
- Dried dill weed: ½ tsp
- Sweet onion, sliced: ½
- Romaine leaves, torn: 4 cups
- Low Fat yogurt: ½ cup

Serves	4
cholesterol	1.97 mg
Calories	125
Sodium	212.14mg
fat	7.65 g
Saturated fat	1.43 g
Dietary fibre	2.76 g

Instructions

1. Begin by heating your oven to 350°F. Thoroughly wash the beets and lightly scrub them, then trim off their stems and roots. Encase the beets in foil and place them on a baking tray. Roast them for approximately 30-40 minutes or until they are tender. After allowing the beets to cool, carefully remove their skins and cut them into fine slices.

2. In a small dish, blend the beets with oil, vinegar, salt, pepper, and dill. In a larger bowl, toss the seasoned beet greens with romaine lettuce and onions. Add small scoops of yogurt atop each portion for immediate

serving.

Crisp Jicama and Red Lettuce Salad

The crunchy sweetness of jicama lends a refreshing contrast to this salad.

- **Jicama: ½ pound**
- **Red lettuce, shredded: 1 head**
- **Radicchio, thinly sliced: 1 head**
- **Red onion, thinly sliced: ½**
- **Balsamic Vinaigrette: ½ cup**

Serves	4
cholesterol	0.1 mg
Calories	208.72
Sodium	99.67 mg
fat	17. 01 grams
Saturated fat	2.24 grams
Dietary fibre	6.12 grams

Instructions

1. Combine jicama with red lettuce, radicchio, and red onion in a spacious salad bowl. Sprinkle with balsamic vinaigrette right before serving.

Warm New Potato Salad

- New potatoes: 2 pounds
- Apple cider vinegar: ¼ cup
- Sugar: 1 tsp
- Olive oil: ¼ cup
- Plain yogurt: ½ cup
- Salt: ¼ tsp
- Pepper: ¼ tsp
- Mustard: 2 tbsp
- Fresh dill weed: 1 tsp
- Sweet onion, finely chopped: ½ cup
- Celery stalks, chopped: 2
- Red bell pepper, chopped: 1

Serves	6
cholesterol	1.12 mg
Calories	254.01
Sodium	100. 1 mg
fat	9.81 g
Saturated fat	1.71 g
Dietary fibre	3. 92 g

Instructions

1. Wash and slice the potatoes into half-inch pieces. Boil them in a large pot of cold water until tender, which should take about 8-12 minutes. Drain the potatoes.

2. While the potatoes are boiling, whisk together vinegar, sugar, olive oil, yogurt, salt, pepper, mustard, and dill in a large bowl. Add the warm, drained potatoes to the bowl and toss to coat. Then, mix in onions, celery, and bell peppers. Chill for 2-4 hours or serve right away.

Hearty Wheat Berry Salad

This robust salad features wheat berries as the primary ingredient and is a favorite for those seeking a filling option. Wheat berries are available in bulk at health food stores.

- **Wheat berries: 1 cup**
- **Water: 3 cups**
- **Broccoli florets: 2 cups**
- **Olive oil: ¼ cup**
- **Mustard: 3 tbsp**
- **Plain yogurt: ½ cup**
- **Lemon juice: 2 tbsp**
- **Pepper: 1 tsp**
- **Dried cranberries: ½ cup**
- **Green onions, chopped: 4**

Serves	6
cholesterol	1.47 mg
Calories	301
Sodium	137.01 mg
fat	10.12 grams
Saturated fat	1.70 grams
Dietary fibre	9.02 grams

Instructions

1.1. Rinse the wheat berries, drain them, and cook in a large saucepan with water. Bring to a boil, then cover, reduce heat to low, and simmer until they are tender, which should take about 55-65 minutes. Add broccoli florets, cover to steam for an additional five minutes, then drain.

2. In a larger bowl, whisk together olive oil, mustard, yogurt, lemon juice, and pepper. Add cranberries, wheat berries, green onions, and steamed broccoli, and mix gently. Chill for 3-4 hours before serving.

Pasta Salad with Crisp Vegetables

This salad bursts with the freshness of raw vegetables and is dressed in a zesty vinaigrette, making it a perfect side dish.

- Low Fat mayonnaise: ½ cup
- Olive oil: 1 cup
- White Wine vinegar: ¼ cup
- Garlic cloves, minced: 2
- Fresh oregano, chopped: 1 tsp
- Flat Leaf parsley, chopped: ¼ cup
- Pepper: ½ tsp
- Red bell peppers, chopped: 2
- Celery stalks, chopped: 4
- Yellow summer squash, chopped: 1
- Grape tomatoes (1 pint)
- Whole Grain rotini pasta (16-ounce package): 1 package

Serves	8
cholesterol	0.1 mg
Calories	367.41
Sodium	142.69 mg
fat	14. 76 grams
Saturated fat	2.36 grams
Dietary fibre	1.78 grams

Instructions

1. 1. Boil a large pot of water. In a large bowl, whisk together mayonnaise, olive oil, vinegar, garlic, oregano, parsley, and pepper.

2. Combine bell peppers, celery, squash, and tomatoes with the dressing mixture. Cook pasta as per the package instructions until al dente, drain, and incorporate into the salad. Toss gently to coat and refrigerate for four hours.

➡ Whole-Grain Pasta Alternative

- For those reducing simple carbs, whole-grain pasta is a superior choice to reintegrate pasta into your meals. These are readily available in grocery stores and have a fuller flavor than regular pasta. You might consider blending them with regular pasta initially to gradually introduce the taste to your family.

French-Style Lentil Rice Salad

- Lemon juice: 3 tbsp
- White Wine vinegar: 1 tbsp
- Sesame oil: 1 tbsp
- Olive oil: ¼ cup
- Low Fat mayonnaise: ½ cup
- Curry powder: 1 to 2 tbsp
- Pepper: ½ tsp
- Green onions, sliced: 4
- Flat Leaf parsley, chopped: ¼ cup
- Lentils (16-ounce package): 1 package
- Brown rice: 1 cup
- Red bell peppers, chopped: 2
- Red onion, chopped: ½ cup

Serves	8-10
cholesterol	0.1 mg
Calories	348.54
Sodium	67.53 mg
fat	11.78 grams
Saturated fat	1.74 grams
Dietary fibre	16.98 grams

Instructions

1. In a large bowl, whisk together lemon juice, vinegar, sesame oil, olive oil, mayonnaise, curry powder, pepper, onions, and parsley; refrigerate the mixture.

2. Wash lentils and prepare them as indicated on the package. Cook rice following package directions concurrently. Once both are ready, combine them with the refrigerated mayonnaise blend, adding bell peppers and onion.

3. Stir to ensure all ingredients are evenly coated. Place in the refrigerator,

ensuring it is covered, and allow to chill for a period of 2 to 4 hours before serving.

Low-Fat Red Bean Salad with Taco Chips

Opt for low-fat, whole-grain taco chips to pair with this dish.

- Lime juice: ¼ cup
- Low Fat sour cream: ½ cup
- Plain yogurt: ½ cup
- Crushed red pepper flakes: ½ tsp
- Red onion, chopped: 1
- Jalapeño peppers, minced: 2
- Green bell pepper, chopped: 1
- Celery stalks, chopped: 3
- Beans for Soup: 4 cups
- Shredded lettuce: 6 cups
- Pumpkin seeds: ½ cup
- Crushed low fat taco chips: 2 cups

Serves	6
cholesterol	11.03 mg
Calories	341.27
Sodium	206. 78 mg
fat	9.89 grams
Saturated fat	2.77 grams
Dietary fibre	14.42 grams

Instructions

1. In a large bowl, whisk together lemon juice, vinegar, sesame oil, olive oil, mayonnaise, curry 1. Combine lime juice, sour cream, yogurt, pepper flakes, onion, and jalapeños in a large bowl. Incorporate bell pepper, celery, and beans, mixing thoroughly. Refrigerate until it's time to serve.

2. For serving, lay lettuce on a platter, top with the bean mixture, garnish with pumpkin seeds and crushed taco chips, and serve promptly. powder, pepper, onions, and parsley; refrigerate the mixture.

Crab and Edamame Salad with Surimi

This salad's key ingredient is Surimi, a seasoned and colored imitation crab meat, offering a delightful flavor.

- Olive oil: ¼ cup (divided)
- Shallots, minced: 6
- White Wine vinegar: 2 tbsp
- Dijon mustard: 2 tbsp
- Crushed red pepper flakes: ¼ tsp
- Flat Leaf parsley, chopped: 2 tbsp
- Frozen surimi, thawed: 2 (8 ounce) packages
- Frozen edamame: 1 (12 ounce) package
- Red leaf lettuce, torn: 4 cups
- Curly endive, torn: 2 cups

Serves	4
cholesterol	34.90 mg
Calories	388.67
Sodium	273.14 mg
fat	21.42 grams
Saturated fat	3.03 grams
Dietary fibre	5.32 grams

Instructions

1. Warm a tablespoon of olive oil in a small saucepan over medium heat. Sauté shallots until they become soft, about 3-4 minutes, then transfer to a serving bowl.

2. Add the remaining olive oil, vinegar, mustard, pepper flakes, and parsley to the shallots; whisk to blend.

3. Tear the surimi into bite-sized pieces and incorporate them into the

imxture. Prepare edamame as directed on the package, drain, and add to the bowl. Toss gently to coat.

4. Add the lettuce and endive, toss, and serve straight away. If not served immediately, refrigerate the surimi blend for up to 4 hours and toss with the greens just before serving.

Apple Coleslaw

- Plain yogurt: 1 cup
- Low Fat mayonnaise: ¼ cup
- Buttermilk: ¼ cup
- Mustard: 2 tbsp
- Lemon juice: 2 tbsp
- Fresh tarragon leaves, chopped: 1 tbsp
- Granny Smith apples, chopped: 2
- Red cabbage, shredded: 3 cups
- Green cabbage, shredded: 3 cups
- Walnut pieces, toasted: ½ cup

Serves	6
cholesterol	2.91 mg
Calories	188.32
Sodium	188.36 mg
fat	10.64 grams
Saturated fat	1.36 grams
Dietary fibre	4 grams

Instructions

1. Blend yogurt, mayonnaise, buttermilk, mustard, lemon juice, and tarragon leaves in a large bowl. Add apples, red cabbage, and green cabbage, mixing thoroughly.

2. Place in the refrigerator, ensuring it is covered, and allow to chill for a period of 2 to 4 hours before serving. Top with walnuts before serving.

Citrus Salad

Ideal for warm summer days, this salad shimmers with the addition of lemon-lime soda.

- **Orange Flavored gelatin: 1 (6 ounce) package**
- **Pineapple tidbits: 1 (20 ounce) can**
- **Mandarin oranges: 1 (15 ounce) can**
- **Lemon yogurt: 1 cup**
- **Lemon Lime soda: 1 (12 ounce) can**

Serves	6
cholesterol	1.13 mg
Calories	151.46
Sodium	44.15 mg
fat	0.39 grams
Saturated fat	0.21 grams
Dietary fibre	1.30 grams

Instructions

1. Put gelatin in a large bowl. Drain the pineapple and oranges, reserving the liquid. Heat 1½ cups of the reserved juice until boiling, then pour over the gelatin, stirring until dissolved.

2. Mix in yogurt, then fold in the drained fruits. Carefully incorporate the soda and pour the mixture into a 2-quart mold or dish. Cover and refrigerate for 4-6 hours until set. Cut into squares to serve.

Black-Eyed Pea Salad

This salad features black-eyed peas, which are high in soluble fiber, known to aid in reducing cholesterol levels.

- Dried black eyed peas: 1 (16 ounce) package
- Water: 8 cups
- Plain yogurt: 1 cup
- Olive oil: ¼ cup
- Dijon mustard: ¼ cup
- Dried thyme leaves: 1 tsp
- Salt: ¼ tsp
- Pepper: ½ tsp
- Green bell peppers, chopped: 2
- Red bell pepper, chopped: 1
- Red onion, finely chopped: 1
- Crumbled goat cheese: ½ cup

Serves	6–8
cholesterol	5.23 mg
Calories	177.89
Sodium	213.12 mg
fat	9.54 grams
Saturated fat	2.43 grams
Dietary fibre	4.36 grams

Instructions

1. Wash the peas, drain them, and soak them in cold water in a large pot overnight. The next morning, drain and rinse them, then cover with fresh water and bring them to a boil. Reduce heat and simmer for 75-85 minutes until tender.

2. In a large bowl, whisk together yogurt, olive oil, mustard, thyme, salt, and pepper. Add the cooked peas, bell peppers, and red onion. Toss to

coat everything evenly and garnish with goat cheese. Chill for 4-6 hours before serving.

Vegetables

- **Oven-Roasted Citrus Beets**
- **Sautéed Ginger Sugar-Snap Peas**
- **Crispy Fried Green Tomatoes**
- **Herb-crusted Baby Eggplants**
- **Snow Peas with Shallots**
- **Buttermilk Mashed Potatoes**
- **Grilled Corn with Red Peppers**
- **Oven-Roasted Garlic Corn**
- **Cheesy Polenta**
- **Chilled Veggie-Stuffed Tomatoes**
- **Baked Tomatoes with Garlic**
- **Farro Pilaf**

Oven-Roasted Citrus Beets

Packed with folate, which aids in reducing blood homocysteine levels, beets are a nutritious choice.

- **Red beets:** 6
- **Olive oil:** 2 tbsp
- **Lemon juice:** 1 tbsp
- **Orange juice:** 3 tbsp (divided)
- **Salt:** ½ tsp
- **White pepper:** ½ tsp
- **Plain yogurt:** ¼ cup
- **Mustard:** 2 tbsp
- **Grated orange zest:** 1 tsp

Serves	4
cholesterol	1.94 mg
Calories	133.45
Sodium	272.83 mg
fat	7.79 grams
Saturated fat	1.29 grams
Dietary fibre	3.73 grams

Instructions

1. Begin by heating your oven to 375°F. After washing and cutting the beet stems, place them in a baking dish. Combine them with olive oil, lemon juice, and a tablespoon of orange juice. Season with salt and pepper after mixing. Bake for 40–50 minutes until they soften enough to be pierced with a knife.

2. Let the beets cool for half an hour. Combine yogurt, the remaining orange juice, mustard, and orange zest in a bowl. Once cooled, peel the beets, slice off the ends, and cut into ½-inch slices. Arrange them on a serving dish, top with the yogurt blend, and serve.

mixture. Prepare edamame as directed on the package, drain, and add to the bowl. Toss gently to coat.

4. Add the lettuce and endive, toss, and serve straight away. If not served immediately, refrigerate the surimi blend for up to 4 hours and toss with the greens just before serving.

> **Beets**
>
> - The vibrant red pigment betacyanin found in beets is useful as a dye or natural coloring. Beet greens, which are often thrown away, are highly nutritious and can be prepared similarly to spinach, imparting a pinkish color.

Sautéed Ginger Sugar-Snap Peas

- **Sugar Snap peas: 1 pound**
- **Olive oil: 2 tbsp**
- **Garlic cloves, minced: 3**
- **Fresh ginger root, grated: 1 tbsp**
- **Salt: ½ tsp**
- **Pepper: ½ tsp**
- **Pistachios, chopped: ¼ cup**

Serves	3
cholesterol	0.01 mg
Calories	121.55
Sodium	77.41 mg
fat	12 grams
Saturated fat	1.68 grams
Dietary fibre	1.26 grams

Instructions

1. After washing and draining the peas, warm the oil in a skillet over medium flame. Add the peas, garlic, and ginger; sauté for 3–4 minutes until they're just tender. Season with salt, pepper, and pistachios, then serve promptly.

Crispy Fried Green Tomatoes

- **Green tomatoes: 4 large**
- **Egg: 1**
- **Buttermilk: ¼ cup**
- **Cornmeal: ½ cup**
- **All Purpose flour: ½ cup**
- **Baking powder: 1 tsp**
- **White pepper: ½ tsp**
- **Canola oil: ¼ cup**

Serves	2
cholesterol	27.62 mg
Calories	120.06
Sodium	77.02 mg
fat	3.52 grams
Saturated fat	0.47 grams
Dietary fibre	1.76 grams

Instructions

1. Cut the tomatoes into ½-inch slices and blot dry. Mix egg and buttermilk in a bowl. Combine cornmeal, flour, baking powder, and pepper on a plate.

2. Warm oil in a skillet over medium heat until it reaches 375°F. Coat tomato slices in the egg mixture, then in the cornmeal mix. Fry in batches, flipping once, until each side is golden brown, roughly 3–6 minutes. Drain on paper towels and serve hot.

➡ Pan-Frying

- This dry-heat cooking technique removes moisture from food. Using properly heated oil (375°F) helps to minimize the absorption of fat, with food absorbing about 10% of the oil.

Herb-crusted Baby Eggplants

Baby eggplants are known for their tenderness and come in shades like purple, mauve, and white.

- **Baby eggplants: 8**
- **Salt: ½ tsp**
- **White pepper: ½ tsp**
- **Garlic clove, minced: 1**
- **Lemon zest, grated: 1 tbsp**
- **Dried breadcrumbs: ¼ cup**
- **Parmesan cheese, grated: 2 tbsp**
- **Olive oil: 2 tbsp**

Serves	2
cholesterol	2.83 mg
Calories	184.53
Sodium	175.15 mg
fat	8.63 grams
Saturated fat	1.72 grams
Dietary fibre	6.11 grams

Instructions

1. Heat your oven to 450°F. Score the cut side of halved eggplants with a fork and place them on a baking sheet.

2. Combine salt, pepper, garlic, zest, breadcrumbs, and Parmesan in a bowl. Drizzle with olive oil, mix, and divide among the eggplant halves.

3. Bake for 10–15 minutes until the eggplants are soft and the topping is golden. Serve immediately.

Eggplant

- Eggplants have a mild taste and are often found with purple skin. Baby eggplants are smaller and less bitter than the larger ones. They are low in calories and high in fiber, with a cup offering 2 grams of fiber and about 21 calories.

Snow Peas with Shallots

- Snow peas: 1 pound
- Olive oil: 2 tbsp
- Shallots, minced: 4
- Cremini mushrooms, sliced: ½ pound
- Sherry vinegar: 2 tbsp
- Lemon juice: 1 tsp

Serves	
cholesterol	0.1 mg
Calories	145.38
Sodium	9.84 mg
fat	8 grams
Saturated fat	1.78 grams
Dietary fibre	4.48 grams

Instructions

1. Prepare the snow peas by trimming the ends and removing the strings if necessary. Heat olive oil in a saucepan over a medium flame. Add shallots, snow peas, and mushrooms.

2. Sauté for 3–5 minutes until the veggies are just tender. Mix in vinegar and lemon juice, remove from heat, and serve at once.

Buttermilk Mashed Potatoes

These mashed potatoes have a creamy, butter-like flavor without the actual use of butter.

- Yukon Gold potatoes: 2 pounds
- Olive oil: 2 tbsp
- Buttermilk: ¼ cup
- Low fat sour cream: ¼ cup
- Dijon mustard: 2 tbsp
- White pepper: ½ tsp
- Salt: ½ tsp

Serves	
cholesterol	4.54 mg
Calories	212
Sodium	145. 84 mg
fat	6.16 grams
Saturated fat	1.56 grams
Dietary fibre	3.49 grams

Instructions

1. Chop potatoes into 1-inch chunks. Boil in a large pot, then simmer under a lid until soft, about 25 minutes. Drain and return to the pot.

2. Over low heat, shake the pot to dry the potatoes. Crush them with a fork, then mix in olive oil. Add buttermilk, sour cream, mustard, pepper, and salt, mashing until they're blended, leaving some chunks if preferred. Serve hot.

➡ Potatoes: To Peel or Not?

- Keeping the skins on potatoes adds texture and nutrients. Yukon Gold potatoes have a high viamin A and potassium content, making them a healthy choice.

Grilled Corn with Red Peppers

This colorful side dish is perfect for outdoor grilling, complementing grilled meats or fish.

- **4 ears of fresh corn**
- **Olive oil: 1 tbsp**
- **Onion, chopped: 1**
- **Garlic cloves, minced: 3**
- **Red bell pepper, chopped: 1**
- **Salt: ½ tsp**
- **Pepper: ½ tsp**
- **Cumin: ½ tsp**

Serves	4
cholesterol	0.1 mg
Calories	180.2
Sodium	97.65 mg
fat	5.25 grams
Saturated fat	0.73 grams
Dietary fibre	4.63 grams

Instructions

1. Prepare the grill. Dehusk the corn and grill it 6 inches from the coals for 3-5 minutes, turning often, until it's slightly charred. Let it cool for 10 minutes, then strip the kernels from the cob.

2. Set a saucepan on the grill, heat olive oil, and sauté onion and garlic until soft, about 5 minutes. Add bell pepper and corn; sauté for 2 more minutes. Season with salt, pepper, and cumin, stir and serve.

Oven-Roasted Garlic Corn

Roasting corn intensifies its sweetness and adds a chewy texture.

- Frozen corn, thawed: 3 cups
- Olive oil: 2 tbsp
- Shallots, minced: 2
- Roasted garlic, from 1 head
- Salt: ½ tsp
- White pepper: ½ tsp

Serves	6
cholesterol	0.1 mg
Calories	150.66
Sodium	81.63 mg
fat	7.10 grams
Saturated fat	0.84 grams
Dietary fibre	2.23 grams

Instructions

1. Heat your oven to 425°F. Pat the corn dry. Position a silicone mat atop a baking tray. Mix corn, olive oil, and shallots on the pan, then spread evenly.
2. Roast for 14-22 minutes, stirring once, until the corn turns a light golden brown.
3. Mix in roasted garlic cloves, salt, and white pepper. Stir well and serve.

Cheesy Polenta

Polenta, a traditional Italian dish, can be enhanced with fresh herbs, sautéed veggies, or various cheeses.

- **Salt: ¼ tsp**
- **Water: 3 cups**
- **Skim milk: 1 cup**
- **Yellow cornmeal: 1¼ cups**
- **plant sterol margarine: 1 tbsp**
- **Parmesan cheese, grated: ¼ cup**
- **Havarti cheese, shredded: ¼ cup**
- **Crushed red pepper flakes: ½ tsp**

Serves	6
cholesterol	14 mg
Calories	173.45
Sodium	214.86 mg
fat	4.99 grams
Saturated fat	2.85 grams
Dietary fibre	2.13 grams

Instructions

1. Boil salted water in a large pot. Mix milk and cornmeal in a bowl until smooth.

2. Gradually whisk the cornmeal mix into the boiling water. Cook on medium-low, stirring constantly, until thick, about 5-10 minutes. Incorporate the margarine, various cheeses, and crushed red pepper flakes. Serve immediately.

Chilled Veggie-Stuffed Tomatoes

This refreshing side can also serve as a vegetarian main course, especially when paired with fruit salad and seed breadsticks.

- **Olive oil: 1 tbsp**
- **Onion, chopped: 1**
- **Garlic cloves, minced: 3**
- **Green bell pepper, chopped: 1**
- **Celery stalks, chopped: 4**
- **Fresh chives, chopped: 1 tbsp**
- **Fresh oregano leaves: 2 tsp**
- **Salt: ½ tsp**
- **Pepper: ½ tsp**
- **Plain yogurt: ½ cup**
- **Lime juice: 1 tbsp**
- **Parmesan cheese, grated: 2 tbsp**
- **Tomatoes, large: 4**

Serves	4
cholesterol	6.42 mg
Calories	112.13
Sodium	199.47 mg
fat	6 grams
Saturated fat	1.74 grams
Dietary fibre	4.18 grams

Instructions

1. Warm olive oil in a saucepan over medium heat. Sauté onion, garlic, and green bell pepper until crisp-tender, about 4 minutes. Off the heat, add celery, chives, oregano, salt, and pepper. Blend the margarine, assorted cheeses, and red pepper flakes.

2. Combine the yogurt, lime juice, and Parmesan cheese with the cooled mix of vegetables. Slice off the tops of the tomatoes and carefully remove the inner flesh and seeds to create a shell approximately half an inch thick.

Fill these tomato shells with the prepared vegetable blend. Refrigerate, covered, for two to three hours before serving.

Baked Tomatoes with Garlic

Baked tomatoes become succulent and rich, pairing well with garlic and cheese.

- **Garlic cloves, minced: 4**
- **Fresh basil, chopped: 3 tbsp**
- **Dried breadcrumbs: 6 tbsp**
- **Pepper: ½ tsp**
- **Fontina cheese, shredded: ¼ cup**
- **Olive oil: 2 tbsp**
- **Plum tomatoes: 6**

Serves	6
cholesterol	17.69 mg
Calories	130.11
Sodium	163.71 mg
fat	9.15 grams
Saturated fat	3.61 grams
Dietary fibre	0.84 grams

Instructions

1. Warm the oven to 400°F. Mix garlic, basil, breadcrumbs, pepper, and Fontina with olive oil.

2. Slice tomatoes in half lengthwise and place them on a parchment-lined baking sheet. Top with the breadcrumb mix.

3. Bake for 12-15 minutes until the tomatoes are tender and the topping is golden. Serve hot.

Farro Pilaf

For a faster alternative, replace farro with spelled or quinoa, following the package instructions for cooking.

- **Farro: 1½ cups**
- **Olive oil: 2 tbsp**
- **Onion, chopped: 1**
- **Garlic cloves, minced: 4**
- **Shredded carrots: 1 cup**
- **Dry white wine: ¼ cup**
- **Salt: ½ tsp**
- **Pepper: ½ tsp**

Serves	6
cholesterol	0.1 mg
Calories	225.81
Sodium	64.09 mg
fat	5.49 grams
Saturated fat	0.79 grams
Dietary fibre	6.69 grams

Instructions

1. Rinse farro thoroughly and soak in a pot of cold water for 8 hours at room temperature. Boil, then simmer for 1½ to 2 hours until chewy yet tender. Drain if needed.

2. In a separate pot, heat olive oil over medium heat. Cook onion and garlic until crisp-tender, about 4 minutes. Add carrots and the drained farro, sautéing for 2-3 minutes.

3. Pour in wine, season with salt and pepper, and simmer until the wine is mostly absorbed. Stir well and serve hot.

Farro

- an ancient grain first grown by Egyptians, farro is a wheat ancestor. It has a nutty flavor and chewy texture, requires soaking, and is rich in fiber, protein, vitamins, and minerals.

Appetizer, snacks and beverages

- **Spicy Roasted Red Bell Pepper Dip**
- **Vanilla and Sweet Spice Dip with Dried Plums and Pecans**
- **Fresh Basil and Kalamata Hummus**
- **Zucchini Spread**
- **Nectarine-Plum Chutney**
- **Canapés with Roasted Garlic, Artichoke, and Chèvre Spread**
- **Stuffed Cremini Mushrooms with Kale and Ham**
- **Orange-Strawberry Drink**
- **Pineapple Bliss Shake**
- **Banana Mini Snack Cakes**

Spicy Roasted Red Bell Pepper Dip

- Non-fat sour cream: 1 cup
- Roasted red bell peppers, water-packed, drained: 7 oz jar
- Fresh dill, roughly chopped: ¼ cup
- Garlic powder: ¼ tsp
- Cayenne or crushed red pepper: ¼ tsp
- Smoked paprika: ¼ tsp
- Salt: 1/8 tsp
- Dried minced onion: 3 tbsp

Serves	16
cholesterol	3 mg
Calories	23
Sodium	55.5 mg
fat	0.01 grams
Saturated fat	0.01 grams
Dietary fibre	0.01 grams

Instructions

1. Blend all ingredients except the onion in a food processor or blender until smooth, about 30 seconds. Pour into a serving bowl and mix in the onion. Chill covered for 30 minutes before serving. Stir again before serving.

Smoked Paprika

- Red bell peppers, which have been smoked over wooden planks and subsequently pulverized, transform into smoked paprika, imparting a rich hue and savory taste to an array of dishes, ranging from broths to garnishes.

Vanilla and Sweet Spice Dip with Dried Plums and Pecans

A divine blend of creamy vanilla yogurt, aromatic spices, succulent dried plums, and toasted pecans. Pair with apple slices, strawberries, pineapple, or low-fat gingersnaps for dipping.

- Chopped pecans: 2 tbsp
- Cooking spray
- Light brown sugar: 1 tsp
- Ground nutmeg: 1/8 tsp
- Fat-free vanilla yogurt: 6 oz
- Ground cinnamon: 1/2 tsp
- Ground ginger: 1/8 tsp
- Chopped dried plums: 3 oz

Serves	8
cholesterol	0.01 mg
Calories	59.3
Sodium	17.3 mg
fat	1.7 grams
Saturated fat	0.1 grams
Dietary fibre	0.1 grams

Instructions

1. Place the pecans into a compact frying pan and give them a slight coating of cooking spray. Distribute the brown sugar and nutmeg over the nuts. Heat them on a medium setting for 1 to 2 minutes, or until the sugar has melted and formed a slight caramel glaze on the pecans, stirring without pause. Move the pecans onto a small dish and allow them to cool for approximately 5 minutes.

Take a small bowl appropriate for serving and vigorously mix the yogurt with cinnamon and ginger. Fold the plums into this mixture. if you wish to serve it straight away, garnish the dip with the prepared pecans and serve.

Fresh Basil and Kalamata Hummus

- No-salt-added cannellini beans, rinsed and drained: 15.5 oz can
- Fresh basil, roughly chopped: 1/2 cup
- Non-fat sour cream: 1/2 cup
- Pitted kalamata olives: 12
- Extra virgin olive oil: 2 tbsp
- Garlic clove, minced: 1 medium
- Salt: 1/4 tsp

Serves	14
cholesterol	2.51mg
Calories	60
Sodium	111 mg
fat	4.3 grams
Saturated fat	1.01 grams
Dietary fibre	1.3 grams

Instructions

Blend all components in a food processor or blender until they reach a smooth consistency. Serve in a small bowl.

Zucchini Spread

This versatile spread, rich with nuts, pairs well with salt-free crackers or vegetable sticks

- **Shredded zucchini, moisture removed with paper towels: 3 1/2 cups**
- **Finely chopped parsley or cilantro: 1/4 cup**
- **Red wine vinegar: 2 tbsp**
- **Extra virgin olive oil: 1 tbsp**
- **Garlic clove, minced: 1 medium**
- **Salt: 1/4 tsp**
- **Pepper to taste**
- **Finely chopped walnuts or pecans, dry-roasted: 2 tbsp**

Serves	8
cholesterol	0.1 mg
Calories	36
Sodium	74 mg
fat	2.97 grams
Saturated fat	0.9 grams
Dietary fibre	1 grams

Instructions

1. Blend all ingredients except nuts until smooth in a food processor or blender. Fold in nuts and chill until serving.

➤ Seed Roasting Tip

- Roasting nuts, even in small amounts, enhance their flavor significantly. Spread them in a skillet and roast over medium heat until fragrant, about 4 minutes, stirring often to prevent burning.

Nectarine-Plum Chutney

This sweet chutney is an excellent appetizer when served atop salt-free crackers with a spread of low-fat cream cheese. It's also a delightful condiment for curried dishes or as an accompaniment to grilled or roasted entrees.

- **Small plums, diced: 3**
- **Medium Granny Smith apple, peeled and diced: 1**
- **Medium nectarine, diced: 1**
- **Sugar: 1/4 cup**
- **Small onion, diced: 1/4**
- **Medium red bell pepper, diced: 1/4**
- **Cider vinegar: 1/4 cup**
- **Golden raisins: 2 tbsp**
- **Grated orange zest: 1 tsp**
- **Salt: 1/8 tsp**
- **Ground nutmeg: 1/8 tsp**

Serves	6
cholesterol	3.5 mg
Calories	89.07
Sodium	50 mg
fat	1.09 grams
Saturated fat	2.43 grams
Dietary fibre	2.3 grams

Instructions

Combine all ingredients in a suitable saucepan and cook over medium-high heat until sugar dissolves. Simmer until fruit is tender, about 40-45 minutes. Cool and refrigerate until serving.

Canapés with Roasted Garlic, Artichoke, and Chèvre Spread

- **Medium garlic cloves, unpeeled: 6**
- **Whole-grain pitas, each cut into sixths: 6 (7-inch)**
- **Frozen artichoke hearts, thawed and chopped: 9 oz**
- **Light mayonnaise: 1/2 cup**
- **Soft goat cheese: 2 oz**
- **Pepper (white preferred): 1/8 tsp**
- **Thinly sliced green onions (green part only): 2 tbsp**
- **Cherry tomatoes, halved lengthwise: 18**

Serves	12
cholesterol	4.3 mg
Calories	96
Sodium	213 mg
fat	4 grams
Saturated fat	0.72 grams
Dietary fibre	3.1 grams

Instructions

1 Begin by setting the oven temperature to 350 degrees Fahrenheit. Place the garlic into a suitable garlic roaster or a small dish that is safe for oven use, and set it on the lowermost rack inside the oven. Allow the garlic to roast for a duration of 5 minutes.

2. While the garlic is roasting, lay out the pita breads flat on a cookie sheet, ensuring they do not overlap. Once the garlic has been in the oven for 5 minutes, position the cookie sheet with the pita breads on the central rack

of the oven and continue to bake for an additional 10 minutes. Afterward, remove both the garlic and pita breads from the oven, transferring them to wire racks to cool for 10 minutes. Keep the oven turned on during this process.

3. Next, remove and discard the bottom ends of the garlic cloves. Gently press out the roasted garlic onto a chopping board, leaving behind the skins. Chop the garlic finely and then place it into a bowl of medium size.

4, To the bowl, add chopped artichokes, mayonnaise, crumbled goat cheese, and a pinch of ground black pepper. Mix these ingredients thoroughly. Once baked, serve the pita slices warm and enjoy immediately.

Stuffed Cremini Mushrooms with Kale and Ham

This chic appetizer is sure to impress your guests.

- Olive oil: 1 tbsp
- Diced medium onion: 1
- Minced garlic cloves: 2
- Large cremini mushrooms, stems removed and chopped: 12 (about 14 ounces)
- Roughly chopped baby kale: 2 cups
- Minced low-sodium, low-fat ham: 3 ounces (trim off any fat)
- Whole-wheat panko breadcrumbs: 1 cup
- Fat-free, low-sodium vegetable broth: 1 ½ cups (divided)
- Finely shredded or grated Parmesan cheese: 2 tbsp

Serves	6
cholesterol	8.2 mg
Calories	125
Sodium	176.2 mg
fat	4.2 grams
Saturated fat	1.6 grams
Dietary fibre	3 grams

Instructions

1. Preheat your oven up to 350°F. Grab a large nonstick skillet, drizzle in the oil, and heat it over a medium-high flame. Toss in the onion and garlic and stir them for about 2 minutes until the onion softens.

Add the mushroom stems, kale, and ham, cooking everything until the mushrooms are tender about 3 minutes. Next, add the panko and 1 cup of broth, cook it all together until it's nice and warm, stirring now and then.

2. Now, stuff those mushroom caps with your kale mixture and line them up on a baking sheet. Drizzle the remaining ½ cup broth over the stuffed caps and cover them with foil. Bake them for 20 to 30 minutes until the mushrooms are soft. Just before you're ready to serve, sprinkle them with Parmesan cheese.

Orange-Strawberry Drink

Elevate your morning orange juice with this quick and easy blend of fruits, perfect for a refreshing start to your day.

- **Fresh orange juice: 2 cups**
- **100% apricot nectar: 1 ½ cups**
- **Frozen unsweetened strawberries: 1 cup**

Serves	6
cholesterol	0.02 mg
Calories	84
Sodium	3.4 mg
fat	0.0 grams
Saturated fat	0.0 grams
Dietary fibre	1.3 grams

Instructions

1. Whizz everything in a blender or food processor until it's smooth and frothy, then serve it up right away for the freshest taste.

Pineapple Bliss Shake

Skip the sugary shakes from fast-food joints and whip up this tropical treat in no time. It's a breeze to make and way healthier.

- **Crushed pineapple in juice: 1 can (15.5 ounces)**
- **Fat-free, sugar-free frozen vanilla ice cream or yogurt: 2 cups**
- **Vanilla extract: 1 tsp**

Serves	4
cholesterol	0.01 mg
Calories	151
Sodium	59 mg
fat	0.01 grams
Saturated fat	0.01 grams
Dietary fibre	1.4 grams

Instructions

1. Process it until it's creamy and smooth in a blender, then enjoy your homemade shake.

Banana Mini Snack Cakes

These little cakes are a triple threat with banana, orange juice, and applesauce or strawberries, making them moist and flavorful. They're perfect for snacking, packing in lunches, or grabbing on the go.

- Cooking spray
- White whole-wheat flour: 1 ½ cups
- Light brown sugar, firmly packed: ⅓ cup
- Baking powder: 2 tsp
- Ground cinnamon: ½ tsp
- Baking soda: ¼ tsp
- Salt: ⅛ tsp
- Pureed banana (equivalent to approximately one average-sized banana): 1/2 cup
- Fresh orange juice: ½ cup
- Egg substitute: ¼ cup
- Unsweetened applesauce or diced strawberries: ¼ cup
- Canola or corn oil: 1 tbsp
- Poppy seeds: 2 tsp

Serves	12
cholesterol	4.32 mg
Calories	119
Sodium	132.1 mg
fat	0.01 grams
Saturated fat	0.01 grams
Dietary fibre	2.67 grams

Instructions

1. Preheat your oven to 400°F and give your muffin pans a light spray with cooking spray. Mix the flour, brown sugar, baking powder, cinnamon, baking soda, and salt in one bowl. In another, mix the banana, orange juice, egg substitute, applesauce or strawberries, oil, and poppy seeds. Combine the wet and dry ingredients until just moistened, then spoon the batter into the pan.

2. Bake for 12 to 13 minutes until a toothpick comes out clean. Let them cool for 5 minutes before serving. Store any leftovers in an airtight bag in the fridge for up to five days or freeze them for up to two months.

Soups

- **Hearty Barley Vegetable Soup**
- **Simple Parmesan Pasta Soup**
- **Cajun Gumbo with Greens and Ham**
- **Creamy Broccoli-Cheese Soup**
- **Tomato Soup with Pasta and Chickpeas**
- **Three-Pepper and Bean soup with Rotini**
- **Zesty SpinachSoup with a Lemon Twist**

Hearty Barley Vegetable Soup

This warm and comforting soup is enhanced by the subtle smokiness of cumin, featuring a nourishing mix of whole grains and colorful vegetables.

- **Fat-free sour cream: ¼ cup**
- **Bottled white horseradish, drained: ½ tsp**
- **Dried basil, crumbled: ⅛ tsp**
- **Olive oil: 1 tsp**
- **Celery, chopped: 1 medium stalk**
- **Onion, chopped: ½ medium**
- **Red bell pepper, chopped: ½ medium**
- **Thawed frozen whole-kernel corn: ½ cup**
- **Ground cumin: ½ tsp**
- **Pepper: ¼ tsp**
- **Salt: ⅛ tsp**
- **Fat-free, low-sodium chicken broth: 3 ½ cups**
- **Quick-cooking barley, uncooked: ⅓ cup**

Serves	4
cholesterol	3.8 mg
Calories	128.1
Sodium	153.5 mg
fat	0.34 grams
Saturated fat	0.32 grams
Dietary fibre	4.98 grams

Instructions

1. Combine sour cream, horseradish, and basil in a small bowl. Whisk well, cover, and chill until needed.

2. Heat olive oil in a saucepan over medium-high heat. Sauté celery, onion, and bell pepper for 3-4 minutes until onions soften, stirring often.

3. Add corn, cumin, pepper, and salt, cooking for 1 minute until cumin is aromatic.

4. Pour in broth and barley, bring to a simmer, then lower heat and simmer covered for 10 minutes until barley is soft.

5. Serve garnished with the chilled sour cream mixture.

Simple Parmesan Pasta Soup

This light yet satisfying soup is perfect for all seasons and uses common pantry items. Add diced chicken breast for a heartier main dish.

- **Egg substitute: ½ cup**
- **Fat-free, low-sodium chicken broth: 4 cups**
- **Whole-grain pasta or crushed whole-grain macaroni, dried: 1 cup**
- **Grated Parmesan cheese: ¼ cup**
- **Fresh parsley, chopped: 1 tbsp**

Serves	6
cholesterol	2.57 mg
Calories	97
Sodium	120 mg
fat	0.21 grams
Saturated fat	0.19 grams
Dietary fibre	9.3 grams

Instructions

1. Whisk egg substitute until well blended.

2. In a saucepan, bring broth to a simmer, stir in pasta, and simmer for 10 minutes until tender.

3. Whisk in the egg substitute and cook for another minute.
4. Serve sprinkled with Parmesan and parsley.

Cajun Gumbo with Greens and Ham

This gumbo gains deep flavor from toasted flour, avoiding extra fat from a traditional roux. The classic blend of vegetables, okra, and greens provides an authentic Cajun experience.

- All-purpose flour: ½ cup
- Uncooked brown rice: 1 ¼ cups
- Cooking spray
- Onions, chopped: 2 medium
- Celery stalks, chopped: 2 medium
- One medium-sized bell pepper, either yellow or green, finely diced.
- Red bell pepper, chopped: 1 medium
- Garlic cloves, minced: 6
- Water: 3 cups
- Low-sodium, low-fat ham (fat removed), chopped: 2 cups
- Fresh or thawed frozen okra, sliced: 1 ½ cups
- Chopped greens (collards, mustard, kale, or spinach): 6 ounces
- Watercress, chopped: 2 bunches
- Fresh parsley, chopped: 1 bunch
- Pepper: ¼ to ½ tsp
- Red hot-pepper sauce (to taste): ¼ tsp
- Cayenne: ⅛ to ¼ tsp

Serves	8
cholesterol	19.5 mg
Calories	217
Sodium	346 mg
fat	4.6 grams
Saturated fat	3.6 grams
Dietary fibre	4.3 grams

Instructions

1. Toast flour in a large saucepan or Dutch oven over medium-high heat for 5 minutes, stirring occasionally. Continue on medium heat until browned, stirring constantly. Transfer to a bowl and cool the pan.

2. Cook rice as directed, omitting salt and margarine.

3. Spray cooled pan with cooking spray. Cook onions, celery, bell peppers, and garlic over medium heat for 15 minutes, stirring occasionally.

4. Stir in toasted flour and the remaining ingredients except rice. Heat until boiling, then reduce to a low heat and let cook gently with a lid for 30 minutes.

5. Serve gumbo over rice on your plate.

Creamy Broccoli-Cheese Soup

Enjoy a velvety soup with less saturated fat and sodium, served best with a crusty whole-grain roll.

- **Fat-free, low-sodium chicken broth: 2 ½ cups**
- **Chopped broccoli or frozen chopped broccoli, thawed: 6 ounces or 10 ounces**
- **Carrot, chopped: 1 medium**
- **Celery stalk, chopped: 1 medium**
- **Salt: ¼ tsp**
- **Pepper: ¼ tsp**
- **Ground nutmeg: ⅛ tsp**
- **All-purpose flour: 3 tbsp**
- **Fat-free half-and-half: 1 cup**
- **Low-fat sharp Cheddar cheese, torn or shredded: 3 slices**

Serves	4
cholesterol	5.7 mg
Calories	123
Sodium	375mg
fat	1.78 grams
Saturated fat	2.5 grams
Dietary fibre	2.67 grams

Instructions

1. Combine broth, broccoli, carrot, celery, salt, pepper, and nutmeg in a saucepan. Simmer over medium-high heat until vegetables are tender.

2. Whisk flour into half-and-half until smooth, then whisk into the soup. Simmer until thickened, stirring occasionally.

3. Add Cheddar and remove from heat. Stir until the cheese melts.

➡ For reheating, use a double boiler to prevent scorching.

Tomato Soup with Pasta and Chickpeas

This tomato soup is enriched with pasta and chickpeas, making it a standalone dish or a perfect companion to a low-fat grilled cheese sandwich.

- Olive oil: 1 tsp
- Onion, chopped: 1 small
- Celery stalk, chopped: 1 medium
- Garlic cloves, minced: 2
- Water: 2 cups
- No-salt-added diced tomatoes, undrained: 1 can (14.5 ounces)
- No-salt-added tomato sauce: 1 can (8 ounces)
- Low-sodium Worcestershire sauce: 1 ½ tbsp
- Salt-free instant chicken bouillon packets: 2
- Sugar: 2 tsp
- Dried oregano, crumbled: 1 ½ tsp
- Dried basil, crumbled: ½ tsp
- Pepper: ½ tsp
- Dried whole-grain elbow macaroni: ⅔ cup
- No-salt-added chickpeas or cannellini beans, rinsed and drained: 1 can (15.5 ounces)
- Fat-free half-and-half: ½ cup
- Grated Parmesan cheese: 2 tbsp

Serves	6
cholesterol	3.1 mg
Calories	179
Sodium	131 mg
fat	0.3 grams
Saturated fat	0.67 grams
Dietary fibre	6.4 grams

Instructions

1. Warm the oil in a mid-sized pot over a moderately high flame, ensuring the base is evenly covered. Saute the chopped onion and celery for about 3 minutes until they soften, making sure to stir now and then. Add the garlic and continue to sauté for another half a minute, stirring well.

2. Next, blend the sautéed veggies along with water, whole tomatoes and their juice, tomato puree, and Worcestershire sauce in a food processor or blender until the mixture is nearly smooth, pausing to scrape down the sides once with a spatula. Pour this blended concoction back into the pot.

3. Mix in the bouillon granules, granulated sugar, oregano, basil, and ground black pepper. Heat the mixture until it reaches a rolling boil. Incorporate the uncooked pasta, then lower the heat to let the mixture simmer for 8 to 10 minutes, stirring occasionally, until the pasta becomes al dente.

4. Fold in the chickpeas and cook them up for a minute. After removing the pot from the heat, blend in the light cream. Serve the dish hot, garnished with a generous dusting of grated Parmesan cheese just before Serving.

Three-Pepper and Bean soup with Rotini

Enjoy a bowl brimming with vegetarian goodness, packed with protein and fiber from white beans and whole-grain pasta. This colorful dish includes tomatoes and zucchini, complemented by a convenient blend of frozen bell peppers.

- **No-fat, low-sodium vegetable stock: 2 cups**
- **Frozen mixed red and green bell peppers and onions: 8 ounces**
- **Zucchini, sliced after being halved lengthwise: 1 medium**
- **Cherry tomatoes, cut into quarters: 1 cup**
- **Crumbled dried basil: 1 tbsp**
- **Red pepper flakes: 1/8 tsp**
- **Dried whole-grain rotini: 6 ounces**
- **No-salt-added navy beans, rinsed and drained: 1 can (15.5 ounces)**
- **Olive oil (extra virgin preferred): 1 tbsp**
- **Salt: 1/4 tsp**

Serves	4
cholesterol	0.56 mg
Calories	317
Sodium	174 mg
fat	0.4 grams
Saturated fat	0.8 grams
Dietary fibre	12.1 grams

Instructions

1. In a substantial saucepan or Dutch oven, boil the broth. Add the frozen pepper and onion mix, zucchini, cherry tomatoes, basil, and red pepper flakes. Heat the mixture until it reaches a rolling boil, then reduce the heat to achieve a

steady simmer. Secure a lid on top and allow it to cook for 30 minutes.

2. While the soup simmers, cook the rotini following the package instructions, skipping the salt. Drain thoroughly.

3. Mix the navy beans into the soup, cooking for an additional 5 minutes until everything is warm. Take off the heat.

4. Incorporate the olive oil and salt.

5. Distribute the pasta into serving bowls and pour the hot soup over it.

Zesty Spinach Soup with a Lemon Twist

This vibrant, easy-to-make soup can be a delightful addition to your meal, especially when paired with Mediterranean Grilled Salmon and a side of steamed or sautéed spinach.

- **Fat-free, low-sodium chicken stock: 2 cups**
- **Fresh lemon juice: 2 tsp**
- **Crumbled dried thyme: ¼ tsp**
- **Salt: 1/16 tsp**
- **Spinach or other greens (kale, escarole), torn into bite-sized pieces: 4 leaves**
- **Green onion (green part only), thinly sliced: 1 medium**

Serves	3
cholesterol	0.7 mg
Calories	21.4
Sodium	224 mg
fat	0.6 grams
Saturated fat	0.8 grams
Dietary fibre	9.3 grams

Instructions

1. In a small saucepan, bring the chicken stock, lemon juice, thyme, and salt to a boil.

2. Place the greens in serving bowls. Pour the hot soup over the greens and garnish with sliced green onion.

Fish and Seafood

- **Fish Fillets with Roasted-Veggie Rice**
- **Hearty Fish Chowder**
- **Crunchy Italian Catfish**
- **Grilled Cod with a Creamy Artichoke and Horseradish Sauce**
- **Oven-Baked Flounder with Tomato Crust**
- **Asian-Style Poached Halibut with Broth**
- **Broiled Salmon with Black Olive Pesto**
- **Grilled Salmon with Mediterranean Flavors**
- **Pan-Seared Salmon with Broccoli and Brown Rice**
- **Rotini with Smoky Chipotle Salmon Cream**
- **Tilapia with Lemon-Crumb Topping**
- **Trout with Almonds and Orange-Dijon Yogurt Sauce**

Fish Fillets with Roasted-Veggie Rice

- Yellow summer squash, sliced into ¼-inch rounds: 1 medium
- One medium-sized red bell pepper, sliced into strips approximately 1/4 inch thick.
- Onion, sliced into ¼-inch strips: 1 medium
- Olive oil, divided (extra virgin preferred): 6 tsp (divided)
- Uncooked quick-cooking brown rice: ½ cup
- Fresh basil or parsley, chopped: 2 tbsp
- Grated lemon zest: 1 tsp
- Fresh lemon juice: 2 tbsp
- Cooking spray
- Thin fish fillets (about 4 ounces each), such as sole, flounder, or tilapia, rinsed and patted dry: 4 fillets
- Reduced-sodium seafood seasoning blend: 1 tsp
- Salt: ⅛ tsp

Serves	4
cholesterol	56 mg
Calories	211.5
Sodium	512 mg
fat	9.6 grams
Saturated fat	3.4 grams
Dietary fibre	3.5 grams

Instructions

1. Start by turning on the broiler to preheat it. Prepare a broiler-proof baking sheet by covering it with aluminum foil.

2. Spread the diced squash, sliced bell pepper, and chopped onion onto the prepared baking sheet. Drizzle 2 teaspoons of oil over the vegetables and toss them lightly to ensure they are evenly coated. Lay the vegetables out flat in a single layer.

3. Position the baking sheet approximately 4 inches beneath the broiler and cook for 9 to 10 minutes, or until the vegetables exhibit a nicely browned appearance around their edges. Once roasted to perfection, transfer the vegetables, still on the foil, to a chopping board and roughly chop them.

4. While the vegetables are broiling, proceed to cook the rice as indicated on the package, omitting any addition of salt and margarine.

Fold in the broiled vegetables, fresh basil, and grated lemon zest into the rice once it is cooked. Keep the mixture covered to retain warmth.

5. Prepare the baking sheet again with a fresh sheet of aluminum foil and apply a light coating of cooking spray.

6. Place the fish fillets on the sheet in a single layer. Evenly distribute 2 teaspoons of oil over the fish and season with your chosen spice blend and a pinch of salt.

7. Broil the fish, keeping it 4 inches from the heat source, for about 5 minutes, or until it is cooked through and can be easily flaked with a fork.

8. To serve, plate the fish alongside the herbed vegetable rice. Just before serving, enhance the fish with a splash of lemon juice and a final drizzle of the remaining 2 teaspoons of oil.

Hearty Fish Chowder

- Light tub margarine: 3 tbsp
- Onions, diced: 2 medium
- Button mushrooms, sliced: 1 cup
- Green bell pepper, chopped: 1 cup
- All-purpose flour: ½ cup
- Fat-free milk: 4 cups
- Firm white fish fillets, such as halibut, coarsely chopped: 1 pound
- Fresh parsley, chopped: ¼ cup
- Low-sodium tamari sauce: 1 tbsp
- Freshly ground pepper to taste
- Yukon gold potatoes, peeled, cubed, and cooked until tender: 2 medium
- Dry sherry or 100% apple cider: ½ cu

Serves	6
cholesterol	43.7 mg
Calories	271
Sodium	276mg
fat	4.5 grams
Saturated fat	0.5 grams
Dietary fibre	3 grams

Instructions

1. Melt margarine in a skillet, add onions, mushrooms, and bell pepper, cooking until onions are soft.

2. Stir in flour until blended, then gradually add milk, stirring to a smooth consistency. Bring to a boil with fish, parsley, tamari, and pepper, then simmer for 10 minutes.

3. Add potatoes and sherry, heating the chowder through. When well cooked, serve.

- - Use tamari instead of soy sauce for a richer, gluten-free option.
- - Choose dry sherry for cooking sherry to avoid extra sodium.

Crunchy Italian Catfish

Create your own low-sodium breadcrumbs for this Crunchy Italian Catfish, and pair it with Roasted Brussels Sprouts for a simultaneous cooking experience.

- **Cooking spray**
- **Catfish fillets (about 4 ounces each), rinsed and patted dry: 4**
- **Lemon: ½ (for juice), 1 tsp grated lemon zest, and 1 lemon cut into wedges**
- **Reduced-calorie whole-grain bread (lowest sodium available), torn: 3 slices**
- **Fresh parsley, chopped: 2 tbsp**
- **Parmesan cheese, shredded or grated: 1 tbsp**
- **Dried oregano, crumbled: 1 tsp**
- **Cayenne pepper: ⅛ tsp**
- **Salt: ⅛ tsp**
- **Olive oil: 2 tbsp**

Serves	4
cholesterol	64.7 mg
Calories	212
Sodium	230 mg
fat	17.9 grams
Saturated fat	3.1 grams
Dietary fibre	4.6 grams

Instructions

1. Preheat the oven to 400°F and prepare a foil-lined baking sheet with cooking spray.

2. Arrange fish on the baking sheet, squeeze lemon juice over the top.

3. Blend bread in a food processor to make crumbs, then mix with parsley, Parmesan, lemon zest, oregano, cayenne, and salt.

Combine with oil and sprinkle over the fish.

4. Bake for 12 to 15 minutes until the fish flakes easily. Serve with lemon wedges.

Grilled Cod with a Creamy Artichoke and Horseradish Sauce

- Light margarine: 1 tbsp
- Shallots or onion, finely chopped: ½ cup
- Garlic, minced: 2 cloves
- All-purpose flour: 2 tbsp
- Salt: pinch
- Pepper: pinch
- Fat-free evaporated milk: 1 can (12 ounces)
- Frozen artichoke hearts, thawed, drained, and cut in halves: 9 ounces
- Fresh or bottled white horseradish, drained: 1 to 2 tbsp
- Fresh oregano, chopped, or dried oregano, crumbled: 1 tbsp fresh or 1 tsp dried
- Cooking spray
- Cod or halibut fillets (about 4 ounces each), rinsed and dried: 4 fillets

Serves	4
cholesterol	53.4 mg
Calories	235
Sodium	289 mg
fat	4.0 grams
Saturated fat	0.5 grams
Dietary fibre	6.7 grams

Instructions

1. In a saucepan, melt margarine over medium heat, coating the bottom. Sauté shallots and garlic for 5 minutes until soft, stirring occasionally.

2. Mix in flour, salt, and pepper.

3. Gradually add milk, whisking constantly. Cook for 5-10 minutes until sauce thickens, continuing to whisk. Cook for an additional minute.

Incorporate artichokes, horseradish, and oregano. Cook for another 3-5 minutes until thoroughly heated, stirring constantly. Take off the stove and place a lid on top to retain warmth.

5. Spray grill rack or broiler pan with cooking spray. Preheat the grill to medium-high or broiler.

6. Grill or broil fish for 7 minutes, flip, and continue for another 5-7 minutes until fish flakes easily with a fork
.

7. Serve by spooning sauce over the fish.

Oven-Baked Flounder with Tomato Crust

Enjoy a breadcrumb-crusted flounder, baked with succulent tomato slices, and seasoned with a lemon marinade

- Cooking spray
- Water: 1½ cups
- Fresh lemon juice: 2 tbsp
- Flounder or cod fillets (about 4 ounces each), rinsed: 6
- Freshly ground pepper to taste
- Tomatoes, sliced: 2 large
- Green bell pepper, minced: ½ medium
- Onion, minced: 2 tbsp
- Whole-wheat panko breadcrumbs: ½ cup
- Canola or corn oil: 1 tbsp
- Dried basil, crumbled: ½ tsp

Serves	6
cholesterol	57.3 mg
Calories	163
Sodium	112 mg
fat	6.7 grams
Saturated fat	0.5 grams
Dietary fibre	4.3 grams

Instructions

1. Preheat the oven to 350°F. Spray a 13x9x2-inch baking dish with cooking spray.
2. Mix water and lemon juice in a large dish. Add fish, coat well, cover, and chill for 10 minutes.
3. Drain fish, discard marinade, and place fish in the baking dish. Season with pepper and top with tomato slices, bell pepper, and onion.

3. Combine panko, oil, and basil. Spread over the fish and vegetables. Place in the oven and cook for 10-15 minutes, or until the fish can be effortlessly flaked with a fork.

Asian-Style Poached Halibut with Broth

Dive into the depths of Asian-inspired flavors with a broth that's perfectly seasoned, featuring ginger and a hint of cayenne. The dish is garnished with vibrant carrot confetti for a delightful texture and taste.

- **Fat-free, low-sodium chicken broth: 3 cups**
- **Dry sherry (optional): 2 tbsp**
- **Soy sauce (low sodium preferred): 2 tbsp**
- **Lemon slices: 2**
- **Ginger Root, peeled and sliced: 3 slices**
- **Cayenne: 1/8 tsp**
- **Halibut fillets (about 4 ounces each), rinsed: 4**
- **Green onions (green part only), cut into 1-inch pieces: 5 or 6**
- **Red bell pepper, cut into 1x1/4-inch strips: 1**
- **Celery, cut into 1x1/4-inch strips: 1 rib**
- **Toasted sesame oil: 1/2 tsp**
- **Carrot, grated: 1**
- **Pepper to taste**

Serves	4
cholesterol	58 mg
Calories	158
Sodium	367 mg
fat	3.7 grams
Saturated fat	0.49 grams
Dietary fibre	3 g

Instructions

1. Combine broth ingredients in a wok or large skillet. Cover and heat until boiling.

2. Add fish to the broth, and add to water if needed to cover. Simmer for about 10 minutes per inch of thickness or until the fish flakes easily with a fork. Remove fish with a slotted spatula to serving bowls.

3. Bring broth liquid to a boil again. Add green onions, bell pepper, and celery, cooking for 2-3 minutes until vegetables are tender-crisp. Discard lemon and ginger root.

4. Using a slotted spoon, transfer vegetables to the bowls. Stir sesame oil into the broth and pour into bowls. Top with grated carrot and pepper and serve

Broiled Salmon with Black Olive Pesto

This broiled salmon dish is enhanced with a fragrant pesto made with black olives, orange zest, and citrus, creating a sophisticated flavor profile. It's a quick meal that's rich in omega-3 fatty acids.

- **Cooking spray**
- **Fresh basil, loosely packed: 1 cup**
- **Pine nuts: 2 tbsp**
- **Sliced black olives: 2 tbsp**
- **Grated orange zest: 1 tsp**
- **Fresh orange juice: 2 tbsp**
- **Light mayonnaise: 1 tbsp**
- **Olive oil: 2 tsp**
- **Garlic cloves, minced: 2**
- **Salmon fillets (about 4 ounces each), rinsed and dried: 4**

Serves	4
cholesterol	57 mg
Calories	218
Sodium	152 mg
fat	13.4 grams
Saturated fat	2.5 grams
Dietary fibre	1.3 grams

Instructions

1. Preheat the broiler and spray the broiler pan with cooking spray.
2. In a food processor, blend basil, pine nuts, olives, orange zest, orange juice, mayonnaise, olive oil, and garlic for 15-20 seconds until slightly chunky.
3. Place fish on the broiler pan and spread the basil mixture over both sides of the fish.

4. Broil about 4 inches from the heat for 5-6 minutes, flip, and broil for another 4-5 minutes until desired doneness is achieved.

Grilled Salmon with Mediterranean Flavors

You'll need some time to marinate, but it will be worth it. The fragrant scent of fresh herbs and the zest of lemon transform this salmon into a simple yet delicious dish. Pair it with quinoa or farro and grilled asparagus.

Marinade Ingredients:

- Italian plum (Roma) tomato, finely chopped: 1
- Red wine vinegar: 2 tbsp
- Fresh rosemary, chopped, or dried rosemary, crushed: 1 tbsp fresh or 1 tsp dried
- Fresh sage, chopped, or dried rubbed sage: 1 tbsp fresh or 1 tsp dried
- Olive oil: 2 tsp
- Grated lemon zest: 1 tsp
- Pepper: ¼ tsp

Other Ingredients:

- Six fillets of salmon, each weighing approximately 4 ounces, thoroughly washed.
- Cooking spray

Serves	6
cholesterol	54 mg
Calories	144
Sodium	85 mg
fat	7.3 gram
Saturated fat	2.4 grams
Dietary fibre	0.1 grams

Instructions

1. In a large dish, combine marinade ingredients. Coat the fish with the marinade, cover, and refrigerate for 30 minutes to 2 hours, turning occasionally.

2. Spray grill rack or broiler pan with cooking spray. Preheat the grill to medium-high or broiler.

3. Drain fish, discarding marinade. Grill or broil about 4 inches from the heat for 5-6 minutes, flip, and continue for another 4-5 minutes until fish reaches desired doneness.

Pan-Seared Salmon with Broccoli and Brown Rice

This quick and convenient meal is perfect for a hectic evening, featuring easy-to-prepare brown rice and ready-to-eat salmon.

- Olive oil: 1 tsp
- Garlic, finely chopped: 2 cloves
- Broccoli florets: 12 oz
- Low-sodium, fat-free chicken stock: 1 ½ cups
- Lemon zest, grated: 1 tsp
- Ground black pepper: ¼ tsp
- Uncooked fast-cooking brown rice: 1 cup
- Boneless, skinless pink salmon, flaked: 2 pouches (5 oz each)
- Cherry tomatoes, sliced in half: 1 cup
- Fresh basil, roughly chopped: ¼ cup

Serves	4
cholesterol	25.6 mg
Calories	229.6
Sodium	416 mg
fat	0.2 grams
Saturated fat	2.6 grams
Dietary fibre	4 grams

Instructions

1. Warm the olive oil in a sizable skillet over medium heat, ensuring the base is evenly coated. Sauté the garlic for 10-15 seconds, turning it not to let it burn.

2. Add the broccoli, turn the heat up to medium-high, and cook for 2-3 minutes until it's crisp-tender, stirring now and then.

3. Add the chicken stock, lemon zest, and black pepper. Stir occasionally as you bring the mixture to a simmer.

4. Mix in the rice, then lower the heat and let it simmer with the lid on for 5 minutes. Turn off the heat.

5. Keep it covered for another 5 minutes or until the rice is soft and the liquid fully absorbed.

6. Fold in the salmon, tomatoes, and basil before serving.

Rotini with Smoky Chipotle Salmon Cream

Experience a fiery kick with this seafood pasta, enhanced by chipotle peppers. Pair it with a fresh salad with Gazpacho Dressing for a complete meal.

- **Whole-grain rotini pasta: 6 oz**
- **Green beans, trimmed and cut in half: 12 oz**
- **Fat-free sour cream: ½ cup**
- **Light mayonnaise: ¼ cup**
- **Chipotle pepper in adobo sauce, minced: ½ to 1 pepper**
- **Two teaspoons of adobo sauce, derived from chipotle peppers.**
- **Garlic powder: ¼ tsp**
- **Ground cumin: ¼ tsp**
- **Boneless, skinless pink salmon, flaked: 1 pouch (5 oz)**
- **Fresh cilantro, chopped: 2-3 tbsp**

Serves	4
cholesterol	24.6 mg
Calories	287
Sodium	453 mg
fat	5.9 grams
Saturated fat	1.8 grams
Dietary fibre	7 grams

Instructions

1. Cook the rotini as per the package instructions without adding salt. Add the green beans to the pot 3 minutes before the pasta is done. Drain well.

2. In a large bowl, whisk together the sour cream, mayonnaise, chipotle pepper, adobo sauce, garlic powder, and cumin.

3. Carefully mix in the pasta and green beans.
4. Top with the salmon and cilantro without stirring.

Tilapia with Lemon-Crumb Topping

A speedy alternative to frozen breaded fish, this microwaveable tilapia dish is ready in just minutes, offering a fresh and flavorful option.

- **Salt: ¼ tsp**
- **Tilapia fillets (or other white fish, about 4 oz each), rinsed and dried: 4**
- **Whole-grain crackers, low-sodium: 8 large**
- **Light margarine: 2 tbsp**
- **Fresh parsley, chopped: 1 tbsp**
- **Fresh lemon juice: 1 ½ tsp**

Serves	4
cholesterol	59.6 mg
Calories	165
Sodium	265 mg
fat	5.78 g
Saturated fat	1.67 g
Dietary fibre	1 g

Instructions

1. Season both sides of the fish with salt and place them in a microwave-safe baking dish with a lid.
2. Process the crackers into fine crumbs using a food processor or blender.
3. Melt the margarine in a microwave on medium power for 30 seconds, then stir in the cracker crumbs, parsley, and lemon juice until combined. Sprinkle this mixture over the fish.
4. Cover and microwave on high for 6-7 minutes, or until the fish flakes easily with a fork. Be cautious when uncovering the dish to avoid steam .

burns. Serve.

Trout with Almonds and Orange-Dijon Yogurt Sauce

Enjoy it with Golden Rice and your preferred green veggie.

- Fat-free plain yogurt: ⅓ cup
- Orange marmalade (all-fruit): 1 tbsp
- Dijon mustard (low sodium preferred): 1 tbsp
- Salt-free lemon-pepper seasoning: ½ tsp
- Trout fillets with skin (about 4 ½ oz each), rinsed and dried: 4
- All-purpose flour: 3 tbsp
- Olive oil: 2 tsp
- Almonds, sliced: 2 tbsp

Serves	4
cholesterol	67 mg
Calories	219
Sodium	128 mg
fat	9.4 grams
Saturated fat	1.7 grams
Dietary fibre	1,9 grams

Instructions

1. In a compact bowl, blend the yogurt, marmalade, and mustard until smooth. Seal and store in the refrigerator until it's time to use. Evenly distribute lemon pepper seasoning on the fish's flesh side. Pour flour into a modestly sized, shallow dish. Coat the flesh side of the fish with flour, pressing it in lightly with your fingers to ensure it sticks, then remove any surplus flour before placing the fish on a separate dish.

2. . Next, lightly oil the flesh side of the fish with a pastry brush, then scatter sliced almonds on top, pressing them in softly so they stick to the surface.

3. Heat a large nonstick frying pan and place the fish almond-side down. Sear over a medium-high flame for 3 to 4 minutes per side, or until the fish is cooked through and can be easily flaked with a fork.

4. Before serving, if you prefer the sauce at room temperature, take it out of the refrigerator. After cooking, place the fish skin-side up on a serving dish and let it rest for a minute. Gently remove the skin with tongs, then flip the fish so the almond crust is facing upwards. Present it with the prepared sauce.

Meat

- **Teriyaki-Style Grilled Sirloin**
- **Balsamic-braised beef with Assorted Mushrooms**
- **Sirloin Steak with Portobello Mushrooms**
- **Slow-Cooker Pepper Steak**
- **Bulgur and Lean Beef Bake**
- **Hawaiian Meatballs**
- **Southwestern Beef-Stuffed Pita Tacos**
- **Bean-Enriched Bunless Beef Burger**
- **Pork Tenderloin with Refined Sauce**

Teriyaki-Style Grilled Sirloin

Ignite the grill for a Japanese-inspired teriyaki sirloin steak, garnished with toasted sesame seeds and served with sugar snap peas dressed in toasted sesame oil. Complement the dish with brown rice or additional grilled veggies.

- **Low-sodium soy sauce: 2 tbsp**
- **Dry sherry or white wine vinegar: 1 tbsp**
- **Garlic cloves, minced: 2**
- **ground ginger; ¼ tsp**
- **Light brown sugar: 1 tsp**
- **Toasted sesame oil: 1 tsp**
- **Boneless sirloin steaks (4 oz each), trimmed of fat: 4**
- **Cooking spray**
- **Trimmed sugar snap peas: 6 oz**
- **Water: ¼ cup**
- **Toasted sesame oil: ½ tsp**
- **Dry-roasted sesame seeds: 1 tbsp**

Serves	4
cholesterol	67.2 mg
Calories	184
Sodium	245 mg
fat	7.2 grams
Saturated fat	3.5 grams
Dietary fibre	1.2 grams

Instructions

1. Combine the ingredients for the marinade in a shallow glass container, thoroughly mixing them. Immerse the beef in the mixture, ensuring it is well coated. Seal the container and place it in the refrigerator to marinate for a duration of 15 minutes up to 8 hours, flipping the beef occasionally.

Balsamic-braised beef with Assorted Mushrooms

Slow braising makes this lean beef tender and flavorful, with the liquid forming a delicious sauce. Serve over whole grains like brown rice or farro.

- **Boneless sirloin or eye-of-round steak, fat removed: 1 lb**
- **Mixed mushrooms (enoki, oyster, portobello, shiitake), sliced: 1 lb**
- **Low-sodium beef broth: 1 cup**
- **Balsamic vinegar: 2 tbsp**
- **Fresh rosemary, chopped, 1 tbsp fresh**
- **Onion powder: 1 tsp**
- **Garlic powder: 1 tsp**
- **Bay leaf, dried: 1**
- **All-purpose flour: 2 tbsp**
- **Water: ¼ cup**

Serves	4
cholesterol	66.3 mg
Calories	198
Sodium	73mg
fat	5.3 grams
Saturated fat	1.5 grams
Dietary fibre	2 grams

Instructions

1. use a sizable skillet with a nonstick surface to sear the beef on each side for 2 minutes at a medium-high setting. add the mushrooms and sauté for 2 to 3 minutes until they begin to soften, making sure to stir from time to time. Incorporate the broth, vinegar, rosemary, onion powder, garlic powder, and a bay leaf, ensuring to mix periodically as you bring the mixture to a gentle simmer. Then lower the heat, cover,

and allow it to simmer for 45 to 50 minutes, or until the beef reaches a state of tenderness.

2. In a separate small bowl, combine the flour with water, whisking it to a smooth consistency. Gradually blend this into the simmering beef concoction. Turn the heat up to medium-high and let it cook for an additional 2 to 3 minutes, or until you notice the sauce has thickened, stirring occasionally. Remember to remove and discard the bay leaf before serving.

Sirloin Steak with Portobello Mushrooms

Savory sirloin steak is perfectly cooked and topped with portobello mushrooms and onions in a robust sauce. Pair with low-fat mashed potatoes or a whole grain.

- **Dried thyme, crumbled: 1 tsp**
- **Coarsely ground pepper: ½ tsp**
- **Boneless sirloin steaks (4 oz each), fat removed: 4**
- **Portobello mushrooms, diced: 8 oz**
- **Large red onion, sliced: 1**
- **Low-sodium beef broth: ½ cup**
- **Brandy (optional): 2 tbsp**
- **Dijon mustard, low sodium: 1 tbsp**
- **Worcestershire sauce, low sodium: 1 tbsp**

Serves	4
cholesterol	57.9 mg
Calories	164
Sodium	164 mg
fat	3.5 grams
Saturated fat	3.4 grams
Dietary fibre	2 grams

Instructions

1. Distribute the thyme and pepper evenly on both surfaces of the beef.

2. Place a sizable nonstick frying pan on the stove and warm it at a medium-high setting. Sear the beef for 4 to 6 minutes per side, or until it reaches your preferred level of doneness. Once cooked, move the beef to a serving dish and cover it to retain its heat.

3. Using the same pan, still set to medium-high heat, sauté the mushrooms and onions for 1 to 2 minutes, or until the onions begin to soften, making sure to stir them now and then.

4. Add the rest of the ingredients. Let them simmer for an additional 5 to 6 minutes, or until the mushrooms become tender and the liquid volume has decreased by half, to roughly ⅜ cup, stirring from time to time. Drizzle this mixture over the warm beef and serve.

Slow-Cooker Pepper Steak

- Top round steak, fat trimmed, thinly sliced: 1 lb
- Low-sodium beef broth: 2 cups
- Red bell pepper, sliced: 1
- Green bell pepper, sliced: 1
- Onion, sliced: ½
- Low-sodium soy sauce: 2 tbsp
- Toasted sesame oil: 1 tsp
- Crushed red pepper flakes (optional): ¼ tsp
- Instant brown rice, uncooked: 1 cup
- Cherry tomatoes, whole or halved: 1 cup

Serves	4
cholesterol	62 mg
Calories	263
Sodium	298 mg
fat	5.7 grams
Saturated fat	1.6 grams
Dietary fibre	3.4 grams

Instructions

Combine beef, broth, peppers, onion, soy sauce, sesame oil, and red pepper flakes in a slow cooker. Cook on low for 6-8 hours or high for 2-3 hours. Add rice and cook until tender. Stir in tomatoes before serving.

Bulgur and Lean Beef Bake

Enhance your meal with this hearty casserole that combines the richness of lean beef with the wholesome goodness of bulgur, adding a nutty taste and a boost of dietary fiber. Complement it with a side of Cauliflower au Gratin or your preferred steamed greens.

- Cooking spray
- 1 lb extra-lean ground beef
- 2 medium onions, finely diced
- 4 medium tomatoes, finely diced
- 1 cup uncooked instant or fine-grain bulgur
- 1/2 cup of freshly minced cilantro or parsley
- ½ cup low-sodium vegetable juice blend
- 2 tbsp fresh lemon juice
- 1 tbsp fresh dill weed, chopped, or 1 heaping tsp dried dill weed, crumbled
- ¼ tsp salt
- ⅜ tsp garlic powder
- ¼ tsp black pepper

Serves	4
cholesterol	7.6 mg
Calories	322
Sodium	265 mg
fat	7.2 grams
Saturated fat	2.5 grams
Dietary fibre	10.5 grams

Instructions

1. 1. Preheat your oven to 350°F.
2. Coat a Dutch oven lightly with cooking spray and brown the ground beef over medium-high heat for 4-5 minutes. Stir occasionally to ensure even cooking.
3. Mix in the onions with the beef and cook for another 3-4 minutes until the onions are tender, stirring now and then.

4. Remove from heat and blend in all the other ingredients.
5. Transfer the mixture into a 9-inch square or 11x7x2-inch baking dish.
6. Bake for 15-20 minutes until thoroughly heated.

Hawaiian Meatballs

- Cooking spray
- 1 lb extra-lean ground beef
- ½ cup whole-wheat panko breadcrumbs
- 3 tbsp green onions, finely chopped
- 1¼ tsp garlic powder
- 1¼ tsp ginger root, grated and peeled
- Pepper to taste
- 1 large egg
- 1 cup instant brown rice, uncooked
- 1 8-ounce can pineapple chunks, juice reserved and drained
- ¼ cup brown sugar, packed firmly
- 2 tbsp cornstarch
- ¼ cup white wine vinegar
- 1 tsp low-sodium soy sauce
- 2 medium green bell peppers, sliced into thin strips or rings

Serves	6
cholesterol	72.1 mg
Calories	267
Sodium	243 mg
fat	5.0 grams
Saturated fat	2.0 grams
Dietary fibre	23.3 grams

Instructions

1. Preheat the broiler and lightly coat the broiler pan and rack with cooking spray.

2. In a bowl, combine the ground beef with the rest of the meatball ingredients, except for the egg. Mix gently to avoid overworking the mixture. Incorporate the egg and shape into twelve ½-inch balls. Place on the broiler rack.

3. Broil the meatballs approximately 4 inches from the heat for about 15 minutes until the tops are brown. Flip and broil for

nother 15 minutes until fully cooked. Drain on paper towels.

4. Prepare the rice as per package instructions, omitting salt and margarine.

5. In a skillet, combine the reserved pineapple juice (adding water to make 1 cup) with brown sugar, cornstarch, vinegar, and soy sauce. Cook over medium heat for 3 minutes until the sauce thickens, stirring constantly.

6. Add the pineapple, bell peppers, and cooked meatballs. Place a lid on top, lower the temperature, and allow to gently cook for ten minutes.
7. Serve the rice on plates, topped with meatballs and sauce.

Southwestern Beef-Stuffed Pita Tacos

These delightful pockets, a cross between pita and tacos, are stuffed with taco-seasoned lean beef and fresh vegetables, making them a hit with kids and adults alike. Pair them with Jícama and Grapefruit Salad with Ancho-Honey Dressing and Strawberry Margarita Ice for a complete meal.

For the filling:

- Extra-lean ground beef: 1 lb
- All-purpose flour: 1 tbsp
- Water: 1 cup
- Chili powder: 1 tsp
- Ground cumin: ½ tsp
- Garlic powder: ¼ tsp
- Onion powder: ¼ tsp
- Black pepper: ¼ tsp
- Whole-grain pita pockets, halved: 6 (6-inch)

For the toppings:

- Romaine lettuce, shredded: 1½ cups
- Tomatoes, diced (approximately 1 cup): 2 medium-sized
- Green bell pepper, chopped: ½ cup
- Onion, chopped: ½ cup

Serves	6
cholesterol	42.5 mg
Calories	284
Sodium	389 mg
fat	6.7 grams
Saturated fat	3.1 grams
Dietary fibre	6 grams

Instructions

1. Preheat the oven to 350°F.
2. In a large skillet, brown the beef over medium-high heat for 8-10 minutes. Dust the mixture with flour and blend thoroughly.

3. . Add the rest of the filling ingredients, bring to a simmer, and cook for 3-4 minutes until thickened, stirring occasionally.
4. Wrap pita halves in aluminum foil and warm in the oven for 5 minutes.
5. Fill the pitas with the beef mixture and top with the fresh vegetables.

Bean-Enriched Bunless Beef Burger

These burgers cleverly use beans to substitute part of the beef, resulting in patties that are high in fiber and lower in saturated fat without compromising on their savory beef taste.

- 1 (15.5-ounce) can of pinto beans, (or no-salt-added black) rinsed and drained
- Extra-lean ground beef: 8 oz
- Dry whole-grain breadcrumbs, low sodium: ¼ cup
- Chili powder: 2 tsp
- Ground cumin: 1 tsp
- Garlic clove, minced: 1
- Salt: ¼ tsp
- Black pepper: ⅛ tsp
- Canola or corn oil: 2 tsp
- Fresh cilantro, chopped: 2 tbsp
- Green onion, thinly sliced: 1
- Jalapeño, seeds and ribs removed, minced: 1
- Large tomato, sliced into 4 thick rounds: 1
- Lime, cut into 4 wedges: 1

Serves	4
cholesterol	31 mg
Calories	233
Sodium	221 mg
fat	6.2 grams
Saturated fat	2.2 grams
Dietary fibre	7 grams

Instructions

1. In a bowl, mash the beans slightly with a fork or potato masher. Mix in the beef, breadcrumbs, spices, and seasonings. Shape into 4 burgers.
2. Heat oil in a skillet over medium heat and cook the burgers covered for 4-5 minutes on each side until fully cooked.
3. Combine cilantro, green onion, and jalapeño in a small bowl.
4. Place a tomato slice on each plate, top with a burger, and sprinkle with the cilantro mixture. Serve with a lime wedge.

Pork Tenderloin with Refined Sauce

- low-sodium chicken broth (Fat-free): ¾ cup
- Raspberry or balsamic vinegar: ¼ cup
- Port wine or 100% grape juice: 2 tbsp
- Olive oil: 1 tsp
- Coarsely ground black pepper: ½ tsp
- Dried oregano, crumbled: ½ tsp
- Garlic clove, minced: 1
- Cornstarch: 1 tsp
- Water: 2 tbsp
- fat trimmed, Pork tenderloin sliced into ¼-inch-thick: 1 lb

Serves	4
cholesterol	66 mg
Calories	162
Sodium	68 mg
fat	4.7 grams
Saturated fat	1.8 grams
Dietary fibre	0.01 grams

Instructions

1. Combine broth, vinegar, port, oil, pepper, oregano, and garlic in a saucepan and cook over medium-high heat until reduced by half (to about ½ cup).

2. Dissolve cornstarch in water and whisk into the sauce, cooking on medium heat until thickened.

3. Cook pork in a nonstick skillet over medium-high heat for 3-4 minutes on each side until it reaches an internal temperature of 145°F. Let it rest for 3 minutes before serving with the sauce.

Dessert

- **Pumpkin-Carrot Cake**
- **Chocolate Mini-Cheesecakes**
- **Fresh Peach and Ginger Crisp**
- **Light Baklava**
- **Chocolate Soufflés with Vanilla Sauce**
- **Strawberry Margarita Ice**

Pumpkin-Carrot Cake

Embrace the autumn season with this homemade pumpkin carrot Cake, ideal for a cozy after-school snack or as a sweet addition to lunch boxes.

- **Cooking spray**
- **Finely grated carrots 1 cup**
- **Canned solid-pack pumpkin (not pie filling) ½ cup**
- **Egg substitute ½ cup**
- **Canola or corn oil 1 tbsp**
- **Vanilla extract 1 tsp**
- **White whole-wheat flour 1 cup**
- **Sugar ⅓ cup**
- **Chopped walnuts ¼ cup**
- **Ground cinnamon 1 tsp**
- **Ground ginger 1 tsp**
- **Pumpkin pie spice 1 tsp**
- **Baking soda ½ tsp**

Serves	8
cholesterol	0.01 mg
Calories	146
Sodium	130 mg
fat	4.8 grams
Saturated fat	0.7 grams
Dietary fibre	3 grams

Instructions

1. Preheat the oven to 350°F and lightly coat an 8-inch square metal baking pan with cooking spray.

2. In a medium bowl, combine carrots, pumpkin, egg substitute, oil, and vanilla.

3. In a separate bowl, mix the flour, sugar, walnuts, cinnamon, ginger, pumpkin pie spice, and baking soda.

4. Blend the dry ingredients into the carrot mixture until just combined, with no visible flour.

5. Transfer the mixture to the pre-arranged baking dish and cook in the oven for a duration of 25 to 30 minutes, or until an inserted toothpick in the middle emerges without any residue.

6. Allow to cool on a rack for at least 15 minutes before slicing.

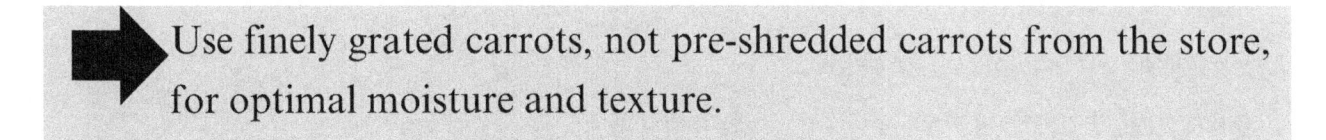

> ➡ Use finely grated carrots, not pre-shredded carrots from the store, for optimal moisture and texture.

Chocolate Mini-Cheesecakes

- **Chocolate graham cracker crumbs ¼ cup and 2 tbsp**
- **Low-fat cream cheese, 4 ounces (softened)**
- **Fat-free cream cheese, softened 4 ounces**
- **Sugar ½ cup**
- **Fat-free sour cream ½ cup**
- **Egg substitute ½ cup**
- **Unsweetened cocoa powder 2 tbsp**
- **Vanilla extract 1 tsp**

Serves	12
cholesterol	9 mg
Calories	95
Sodium	161 mg
fat	2.6 grams
Saturated fat	2.6 grams
Dietary fibre	0.05 grams

Instructions

1. Preheat the oven to 325°F and line a 12-cup muffin pan with foil or paper liners, sprinkling 1½ teaspoons of crumbs into each.
2. In a large bowl, use an electric mixer to blend the cream cheese, sugar, and sour cream until fluffy, about 3 minutes.
3. Incorporate the egg substitute, cocoa powder, and vanilla, mixing until combined.
4. Distribute the mixture into the lined cups, using an ice cream scoop for even portions.
5. Bake for 18-20 minutes until the centers are set. Cool on a rack for 15-20 minutes, then refrigerate for at least 30 minutes before serving.

Fresh Peach and Ginger Crisp

This Fresh Peach and Ginger Crisp, with its sweet and zesty flavor, offers a refreshing twist to the classic fruit crisp.

- **Cooking spray**

<u>Filling</u>

- **Peaches, peeled and sliced 3 pounds**
- **Sugar 2 tbsp**
- **Cornstarch 1½ tbsp**
- **Minced crystallized ginger 1½ tbsp**

<u>Topping:</u>

- **Quick-cooking oatmeal 1 cup**
- **Finely chopped pecans ⅓ cup**
- **Whole-wheat flour ¼ cup**
- **Packed light brown sugar ¼ cup**
- **Ground cinnamon 1 tsp**
- **Minced crystallized ginger 1 tbsp**
- **Fat-free milk 3 tbsp**
- **Canola or corn oil 1 tbsp**

Serves	Serves 6–8
cholesterol	Serves 6–8
Calories	Serves 6–8
Sodium	Serves 6–8
fat	Serves 6–8
Saturated fat	Serves 6–8
Dietary fibre	Serves 6–8

Instructions

1. Preheat the oven to 350°F and lightly coat an 8-inch square baking pan with cooking spray.

2. Mix the filling ingredients and spoon into the pan.

3. In a separate bowl, combine the oatmeal, pecans, flour, brown sugar, cinnamon, and ginger. Gradually add milk and oil, stirring until moistened. Sprinkle over the filling.

4. Bake for 30 minutes until the peaches are tender and the topping is golden. Cool for 30 minutes on a rack and serve warm. Store leftovers in the refrigerator for up to two days.

Light Baklava

- Raisins ¾ cup
- (finely chopped) Dry-roasted pecans or walnuts ⅔ cup
- Butter-flavored cooking spray
- Thawed phyllo dough sheets 8
- Honey ½ cup
- Ground cinnamon 2 tsp

Serves	12
cholesterol	0.04 mg
Calories	164
Sodium	63 mg
fat	0.6 grams
Saturated fat	0.5g rams
Dietary fibre	2 grams

Instructions

1. Start by preheating your oven to 350°F. Mix raisins and nuts in a bowl. Lightly mist every other sheet of phyllo with the cooking spray and stack them up. Spread the raisin-nut mix on the top sheet, leaving an inch free on the edges. Drizzle honey and scatter cinnamon on top. Roll it up from the long side,

2, tuck in the ends, and lay it seam-down on a nonstick baking tray. Mist the top with spray and score the pastry every 1½ inches to let steam escape.

3. Bake for 20-30 minutes until it's a lovely golden brown. Cool slightly and slice into 12 pieces along the scored lines.

▶ If you want to freeze it, prepare everything but don't spray the top or bake. Freeze it solid on a tray, then wrap it for storage. When ready, just spray, bake at 350°F for 35-45 minutes, and enjoy a golden treat!

Chocolate Soufflés with Vanilla Sauce

Indulge in a fluffy chocolate soufflé with a citrus twist and a vanilla sauce that will make you forget about high-fat desserts.

- **Cooking spray**
- **Fresh orange juice ⅓ cup**
- **Sugar ¼ cup**
- **Large egg whites 4**
- **Unsweetened cocoa powder ¼ cup**
- **Orange liqueur or 2 tbsp**
- **frozen yogurt ¾ cup or sugar-free vanilla ice cream**

Serves	6
cholesterol	0.04 mg
Calories	102
Sodium	50 mg
fat	0.04 grams
Saturated fat	0 grams
Dietary fibre	1 grams

Instructions

1. Preheat your oven to 300°F and spritz six small custard cups with cooking spray. Simmer orange juice and sugar in a pan until syrupy, then let it cool. Whip egg whites to stiff peaks, then gently fold in the syrup, cocoa, and liqueur. Fill the cups and bake for 12 minutes until they puff up.

2. Top each soufflé with a dollop of ice cream before serving.

➡ Be careful when separating your eggs, as even a tiny bit of yolk can prevent the whites from reaching the desired peak when beaten.

Strawberry Margarita Ice

This frozen treat borrows flavors from a classic frozen margarita for a refreshing dessert, perfect for a summer barbecue.

- **Strawberries, fresh or thawed if frozen 2 cups**
- **Fresh orange juice ½ cup**
- **Fresh lime juice ¼ cup**
- **Agave syrup ¼ cup**
- **Tequila or lime juice 1 tbsp**
- **Orange liqueur or juice 1 tbsp**

Serves	6
cholesterol	0.07 mg
Calories	81
Sodium	1 mg
fat	0 grams
Saturated fat	0 grams
Dietary fibre	1 grams

Instructions

1. Blend all the ingredients in a food processor or blender until you get a smooth consistency. Then, pour the mixture into a loaf pan measuring 9 by 5 by 3 inches. Wrap it up and pop it in the freezer for about 4 hours. You want it to set until it's firm but not rock hard.

2. While you're waiting, stick a big mixing bowl in the fridge to cool down.

3. Once the mixture is set, break it up into chunks and toss them into

the cold bowl you prepared earlier. Now, grab your electric mixer and whip everything up until it's creamy, but be careful not to let it melt. You can dig in right away or put it back in the loaf pan, cover it, and freeze it until it's time to serve.

If you're ready to serve and it's frozen, just scrape it with a spoon to create fluffy piles, and serve them up in cute dessert dishes or fancy margarita glasses.

> ➡ If you accidentally leave your strawberry mix in the freezer too long and it turns into a block of ice, don't sweat it. Allow it to sit at ambient temperature for approximately 15 minutes. This will soften it enough so you can break it into pieces and beat it as you were supposed to.

Bonus Section

In the next pages, you will find lots of bonuses specifically designed to enhance your journey towards well-being.

We believe these bonuses will complement the wisdom and guidance found within the pages of this book, enriching your experience and empowering you on your journey to optimal health and well-being.

Finally, we humbly request an honest review of this book. Your feedback is priceless to us and if you enjoyed reading this book. we would be grateful if you give this Book a 5-star review.

Thank you!

Exercising

A Fitness Program for lowering Cholesterol

I have many patients who tell me that they hate working out. I tell them it's probably not the right activity for them yet. Like switching to a healthy diet, getting into the exercise habit can be a challenge. One of those habits that needs to be broken is inactivity. You'll know when you've made this switch because you will miss working out on days you don't and crave the good feeling–and occasional soreness–in your muscles that tell you you're getting fitter.

Pros and Cons of Exercising

Exercise has profound benefits for heart health. According to studies, even modest exercise can cut the frequency of heart-related events in half. Aerobic exercise (the kind that raises heart rate) reduces the risk of having a heart attack or stroke by:

- Lowering triglycerides
- Raising HDL cholesterol
- Lowering blood pressure
- Lowering body fat
- Lowering blood sugar
- Lowering mental stress
- Reducing clotting tendency

Exercise increases the pumping capacity of the heart, which means it can push more blood with each beat, delivering oxygen and nutrients to tissues more efficiently. It does this by increasing small blood vessels' ability to supply oxygen to muscles within active areas. Therefore, overall fitness improves as well as endurance; additionally, strength training improves muscle tone while keeping bones strong.

It's never too late! Healthy individuals who begin exercising after age 45 still have about a 23% lower death rate over the next two decades than those who remain sedentary throughout their lives. Even people who've had heart attacks can reduce their chances of having another one through supervised aerobics-based programs – up to 25%. On the other hand, chronic lack-of-exercise doubles the risk for coronary artery disease making it almost as dangerous as hypertension, smoking cigarettes, or abnormal lipids!

Getting Started

If you live a sedentary life, the most important thing to know is that any activity is better than none. Light activities include walking instead of driving or taking stairs instead of elevators; moderate activities involve housework such as cleaning or gardening while vigorous activities involve running/jogging. However, sustained and regular exercise has an even greater impact on health.

Strength training, stretching, and aerobics should all be part of your weekly routine. Aim for at least three sessions per week–one each for strength training (with weights), stretching (yoga), and aerobics (jogging).

Aerobic exercise is best for heart health because it uses large muscle groups in rhythmic/repeating motion over extended periods. Some examples include brisk walking, jogging/running, swimming laps, etc; rowing machine sessions would also count if large muscles are used continuously.

If you have heart conditions, consult your doctor before starting an exercise program. They will provide individualized advice based on your specific situation so that you avoid exceeding limits set by stress tests or causing angina (chest pain).

When done regularly, exercising can cause sprains/strains/shin splints – but don't worry! By choosing low-impact activities; starting slowly & gradually increasing intensity under guidance from healthcare providers who know about these things — you can safely experience numerous benefits including lowered blood pressure; and improved blood sugar regulation leading to healthier hearts overall with fewer complications down the road such as diabetes or stroke among others

Exercise programs require planning and perseverance. The trick is to set up a routine and types of activity that you can stick to over time. Start slowly, set realistic goals, and recognize your achievements. This section includes examples of strength training, flexibility training, and aerobic activity programs. Walking is recommended because it is safe and accessible for most people, including those with heart problems. If you prefer swimming or biking, substitute those activities instead.

Basic Aerobic Training

Walking has now been recognized as a formal type of physical activity. Here's how to start:

Choose a safe place to walk: Consider quiet streets, park trails, school tracks, or shopping malls.

Invest in good shoes: Look for breathable materials like leather or nylon mesh and sturdy but flexible soles with heel elevation.

Find a walking partner or group: While some prefer solitary walks for self-reflection, the company can motivate you and ensure safety.

Dress appropriately by dressing in layers, wearing lighter clothing than usual, and making adjustments as you warm up

Stretch before your walk: Follow the instructions for the 10 essential stretches later in this guide.

Include five-minute warm-up and cool-down periods in your routine.

Continue using proper technique: Keep your back straight, head up, shoulders back and stomach muscles contracted while walking briskly. Lean forward onto the ball of your foot; swing your arms loosely; land on your heels; push off with your toes. When walking briskly or uphill, lean forward slightly and take longer strides at an easy pace.

Increasing Flexibility: Crucial Stretches

Including stretching exercises in your fitness routine is important for increasing flexibility. Regular stretching helps with balance and posture, keeps the body limber, and prevents injury. Each stretch should be done four to five times unless otherwise noted.

Hamstring Stretch

Target: Back of thigh

without leaning back, Sit sideways on a bench. Keep your back and shoulders straight. With one foot flat on the ground, extend the other leg straight out onto the bench. Slowly lean forward at your hips until you feel a stretch in your calf and behind your knee. stay like that for ten- to thirty seconds. Repeat three to five times on each leg.

Calf Stretch

Target: Lower leg muscles

Stand facing a wall with hands on the wall and arms extended. Take a one- to two-foot step back, keeping heel and foot flat on the ground. Stay like that for ten- to thirty seconds. Then bend back leg's knee while keeping the heel flat; hold for an additional 30 to 40 seconds On each leg repeat three to five times

The Triceps Stretch

Target: Back of upper arm

With your right elbow pointing up, bring your right hand towards the back of your neck. Using your left hand, press gently on the raised elbow until you feel a stretch in the triceps. hold for 10 to 30 seconds and do the other hand.

Shoulder Stretch

Target: Upper back and shoulders

Sit comfortably on the front edge of a chair. Raise your arms. Interlock your fingers and lift your arms with your palms facing upwards. Keep looking straight ahead and take back behind your ears. maintain the same position for at least ten seconds to thirty seconds.

Quadriceps Stretch

Target: Front of thighs

Lie on one side with a pillow under your head or hand for support; stack hips on top of one another so that they are in line vertically from top to bottom; bend the top knee until you feel stretch along the front thigh muscle then reach behind grabbing heel if possible (use a towel if necessary). maintain the same position for 10-30 seconds and repeat on the opposite side.

Lateral Stretch

Target: Muscles of the shoulder, side, and trunk

Sit on a chair with a straight back. Extend your right arm upwards and rest your left hand lightly on your left leg. You should feel a stretch in your trunk and ribcage. maintain the same position for ten to thirty seconds. Repeat on the other side.

Dual Hip Rotation

Target: Muscles of the thighs and hips

Lie on your back with feet flat on the ground and knees bent. Keep shoulders down on the ground. While keeping your knees together, slowly lower your legs to one side. maintain the same position for ten to thirty seconds. Return to the center and do the opposite side.

Strength training exercises

Strength training can be a great addition to your fitness routine, although it is not as crucial as aerobic exercise for heart health. Here's what you need to know:

- Aim for two or three 20-minute sessions per week.
- Don't work out the same muscle groups two days in a row.
- Concentrate on arms, shoulders, legs, and torso — these are major muscle groups.

- Start light; increase gradually after getting comfortable with a weight.
- Do each exercise eight to 15 times through; if you get stronger add second or third sets.
- Breathe evenly; move slowly and deliberately.

How Much Exercise Is Enough?

The Surgeon General in 1996, recommended that people burn at least 150 calories per day through exercise — such as walking 1 1/2 miles (roughly). This might seem like a lot at first. Start by walking for what seems like a reasonable amount of time each day — even if it's just 10 minutes — and then gradually add on as it gets easier. Shoot for 30 to 45 minutes of brisk walking or an equivalent amount of activity every day once you have established this habit.

Aerobic exercise should be invigorating but not exhausting; challenging but not debilitating. When you are at an appropriate level of fitness, you should be able to sustain the activity continuously for at least 20-30 minutes. Talking can help gauge intensity: If it is difficult for you to speak, you're pushing too hard; if it is easy for you to sing, you're not pushing hard enough. To prevent injury, always include a five-to-10-minute warm-up and cool-down; starting with a less intense version of your intended activity (such as walking slowly before power-walking) is a great way to do this.

Allocating Time for Exercise in Your Life

How are these new undertakings going to fit into your already booked timetable? I can't add hours to your day, but I can emphasize the significance of making time for exercise. If you need thirty minutes of exercise every day, think about swapping that time with another activity. Should you be watching two hours of TV each night? Could you spend less time on lunch breaks checking emails? Maybe ask a neighbor to join you so that it becomes a social activity too. Be realistic. If you know that after dinner is when you'll be helping the kids with their homework, don't plan exercise around that.

Look for ways to add short bursts of movement and leisure activity throughout the day – like a bike ride on Saturday morning or an extra lap around the mall while shopping. According to studies, dividing your daily 30 minutes into three or four eight- to ten-minute sessions can still benefit cardiovascular health; just make sure they're moderately intense bouts. But avoid doing high-intensity workouts too often.

Make any necessary scheduling adjustments after the first week; the good news is it gets easier as you get used to it!

Tips for sticking with your exercise plans

Setting Goals

For most people, going from a mostly sedentary lifestyle to consistently working out can be tough. Set realistic goals — like losing 25 pounds in a year — and break them into smaller ones, like losing more than two pounds per month. One way to do this is by walking 70 miles a month or taking six 45-minute walks each week.

Tracking Progress

Keep yourself accountable by logging your daily workouts on a chart or in a planner. Seeing how far you've come can be its motivator.

Rewarding Work

When you meet your fitness goals, reward yourself in meaningful ways that don't contradict what you're trying to achieve (so, no doughnuts after running five miles). Instead, treat yourself with something fun that helps move your new healthy lifestyle forward — like splurging on workout gear or buying a new CD for your walks.

Getting Back on Track

Sometimes life gets in the way of even the most dedicated exerciser: work travel, inclement weather, illness, the entire pizza menu at Mellow

Mushroom. Assess where you are physically and adjust your goals accordingly as you get back into the swing of things. Start with shorter workouts until you're used to moving again, then build up from there. Stay positive and focus on how great it feels when you're done sweating ... not during.

Think of something nice to give yourself when you've achieved your first goal after the holiday.

SHOPPING WORKSHEET

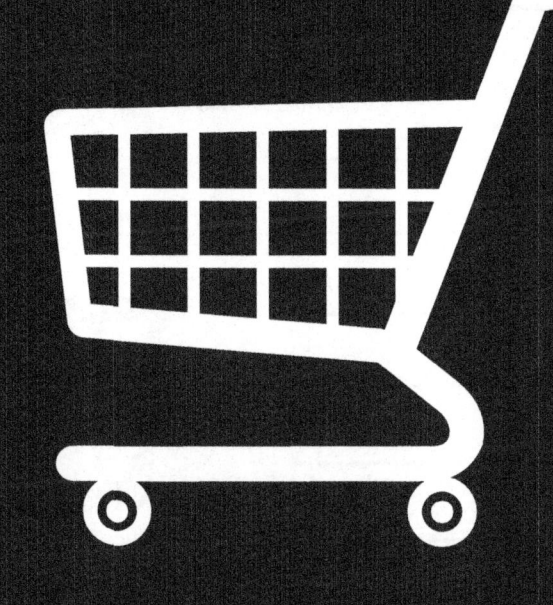

GROCERY SHOPPING LIST

BUDGET: _____

DATE: _____

LIST

☐ _____
☐ _____
☐ _____
☐ _____
☐ _____
☐ _____
☐ _____
☐ _____
☐ _____
☐ _____
☐ _____
☐ _____
☐ _____
☐ _____

☐ _____
☐ _____
☐ _____
☐ _____
☐ _____
☐ _____

GROCERY SHOPPING LIST

BUDGET: _____ **DATE:** _____

LIST

☐ _____ ☐ _____
☐ _____ ☐ _____
☐ _____ ☐ _____
☐ _____ ☐ _____
☐ _____ ☐ _____
☐ _____ ☐ _____
☐ _____
☐ _____
☐ _____
☐ _____
☐ _____
☐ _____
☐ _____
☐ _____

GROCERY SHOPPING LIST

BUDGET: _____

DATE: _____

LIST

- ☐ _____
- ☐ _____
- ☐ _____
- ☐ _____
- ☐ _____
- ☐ _____
- ☐ _____
- ☐ _____
- ☐ _____
- ☐ _____
- ☐ _____
- ☐ _____
- ☐ _____
- ☐ _____

- ☐ _____
- ☐ _____
- ☐ _____
- ☐ _____
- ☐ _____
- ☐ _____

GROCERY SHOPPING LIST

BUDGET: _____

DATE: _____

LIST

- ☐ _____
- ☐ _____
- ☐ _____
- ☐ _____
- ☐ _____
- ☐ _____
- ☐ _____
- ☐ _____
- ☐ _____
- ☐ _____
- ☐ _____
- ☐ _____
- ☐ _____
- ☐ _____

- ☐ _____
- ☐ _____
- ☐ _____
- ☐ _____
- ☐ _____
- ☐ _____

GROCERY SHOPPING LIST

BUDGET: _____

DATE: _____

LIST

- ☐ _____
- ☐ _____
- ☐ _____
- ☐ _____
- ☐ _____
- ☐ _____
- ☐ _____
- ☐ _____
- ☐ _____
- ☐ _____
- ☐ _____
- ☐ _____
- ☐ _____

- ☐ _____
- ☐ _____
- ☐ _____
- ☐ _____
- ☐ _____
- ☐ _____

GROCERY SHOPPING LIST

BUDGET: _____

DATE: _____

LIST

- ☐ _____
- ☐ _____
- ☐ _____
- ☐ _____
- ☐ _____
- ☐ _____
- ☐ _____
- ☐ _____
- ☐ _____
- ☐ _____
- ☐ _____
- ☐ _____
- ☐ _____
- ☐ _____

- ☐ _____
- ☐ _____
- ☐ _____
- ☐ _____
- ☐ _____
- ☐ _____

GROCERY SHOPPING LIST

BUDGET: _____

DATE: _____

LIST

- ☐ _____
- ☐ _____
- ☐ _____
- ☐ _____
- ☐ _____
- ☐ _____
- ☐ _____
- ☐ _____
- ☐ _____
- ☐ _____
- ☐ _____
- ☐ _____
- ☐ _____

- ☐ _____
- ☐ _____
- ☐ _____
- ☐ _____
- ☐ _____
- ☐ _____

GROCERY SHOPPING LIST

BUDGET: _____ **DATE:** _____

LIST

- [ ] _____
- [ ] _____
- [ ] _____
- [ ] _____
- [ ] _____
- [ ] _____
- [ ] _____
- [ ] _____
- [ ] _____
- [ ] _____
- [ ] _____
- [ ] _____
- [ ] _____
- [ ] _____

- [ ] _____
- [ ] _____
- [ ] _____
- [ ] _____
- [ ] _____
- [ ] _____

GROCERY SHOPPING LIST

BUDGET: _____ **DATE:** _____

LIST

☐ _____ ☐ _____
☐ _____ ☐ _____
☐ _____ ☐ _____
☐ _____ ☐ _____
☐ _____ ☐ _____
☐ _____ ☐ _____
☐ _____
☐ _____
☐ _____
☐ _____
☐ _____
☐ _____
☐ _____
☐ _____

GROCERY SHOPPING LIST

BUDGET: _____ **DATE:** _____

LIST

- ☐ _____
- ☐ _____
- ☐ _____
- ☐ _____
- ☐ _____
- ☐ _____
- ☐ _____
- ☐ _____
- ☐ _____
- ☐ _____
- ☐ _____
- ☐ _____
- ☐ _____

- ☐ _____
- ☐ _____
- ☐ _____
- ☐ _____
- ☐ _____
- ☐ _____

WEEKLY FITNESS WORKSHEET

Big results are achieved by doing a little bit every day.

Weekly Fitness

Month : _____

Week: _____

My Motivation

My Weekly Goals

- ☐ _____
- ☐ _____
- ☐ _____
- ☐ _____
- ☐ _____

Notes

Monday Exercises:

Tuesday Exercises:

Wednesday Exercises:

Thursday Exercises:

Friday Exercises:

Saturday Exercises:

Rate your week

★ ★ ★ ★ ★

Weekly Fitness

Month : _____

Week: _____

My Motivation

My Weekly Goals

- ☐ _____
- ☐ _____
- ☐ _____
- ☐ _____
- ☐ _____

Notes

Monday Exercises:

Tuesday Exercises:

Wednesday Exercises:

Thursday Exercises:

Friday Exercises:

Saturday Exercises:

Rate your week

★ ★ ★ ★ ★

My Motivation

My Weekly Goals

- ☐ _____
- ☐ _____
- ☐ _____
- ☐ _____
- ☐ _____

Notes

Monday Exercises:

Tuesday Exercises:

Wednesday Exercises:

Thursday Exercises:

Friday Exercises:

Saturday Exercises:

Rate your week

★ ★ ★ ★ ★

My Motivation

My Weekly Goals

- ☐ _____
- ☐ _____
- ☐ _____
- ☐ _____
- ☐ _____

Notes

Monday Exercises:

Tuesday Exercises:

Wednesday Exercises:

Thursday Exercises:

Friday Exercises:

Saturday Exercises:

Rate your week
★ ★ ★ ★ ★

Weekly Fitness

Month : _____

Week: _____

My Motivation

My Weekly Goals

- ☐ _____
- ☐ _____
- ☐ _____
- ☐ _____
- ☐ _____

Notes

Monday Exercises:

Tuesday Exercises:

Wednesday Exercises:

Thursday Exercises:

Friday Exercises:

Saturday Exercises:

Rate your week

★ ★ ★ ★ ★

My Motivation

My Weekly Goals

- ☐ _____
- ☐ _____
- ☐ _____
- ☐ _____
- ☐ _____

Notes

Monday Exercises:

Tuesday Exercises:

Wednesday Exercises:

Thursday Exercises:

Friday Exercises:

Saturday Exercises:

Rate your week

★ ★ ★ ★ ★

My Motivation

My Weekly Goals

- _____
- _____
- _____
- _____
- _____

Notes

Monday Exercises:

Tuesday Exercises:

Wednesday Exercises:

Thursday Exercises:

Friday Exercises:

Saturday Exercises:

Rate your week

★ ★ ★ ★ ★

Weekly Fitness

Month : _____

Week: _____

My Motivation

My Weekly Goals

- ☐ _____
- ☐ _____
- ☐ _____
- ☐ _____
- ☐ _____

Notes

Monday Exercises:

Tuesday Exercises:

Wednesday Exercises:

Thursday Exercises:

Friday Exercises:

Saturday Exercises:

Rate your week

★ ★ ★ ★ ★

Month : _____

Week: _____

My Motivation

My Weekly Goals

- ☐ _____
- ☐ _____
- ☐ _____
- ☐ _____
- ☐ _____

Notes

Monday Exercises:

Tuesday Exercises:

Wednesday Exercises:

Thursday Exercises:

Friday Exercises:

Saturday Exercises:

Rate your week

★ ★ ★ ★ ★

My Motivation

My Weekly Goals

- _____
- _____
- _____
- _____
- _____

Notes

Monday Exercises:

Tuesday Exercises:

Wednesday Exercises:

Thursday Exercises:

Friday Exercises:

Saturday Exercises:

Rate your week

★ ★ ★ ★ ★

Weekly Fitness

Month : _____

Week: _____

My Motivation

My Weekly Goals

- [ ] _____
- [ ] _____
- [ ] _____
- [ ] _____
- [ ] _____

Notes

Monday Exercises:

Tuesday Exercises:

Wednesday Exercises:

Thursday Exercises:

Friday Exercises:

Saturday Exercises:

Rate your week

★ ★ ★ ★ ★

Weekly Fitness

Month : _____

Week: _____

My Motivation

My Weekly Goals

- ☐ _____
- ☐ _____
- ☐ _____
- ☐ _____
- ☐ _____

Notes

Monday Exercises:

Tuesday Exercises:

Wednesday Exercises:

Thursday Exercises:

Friday Exercises:

Saturday Exercises:

Rate your week

★ ★ ★ ★ ★

Your Bonus

We're excited to offer you a special bonus! Scan the QR code below to claim your free bonus cookbook. As a bonus, you'll also gain access to our exclusive cookbook community, where you can ask questions, share tips, and connect with our team. Don't miss out—just scan the QR code below to get started!

Enjoy and happy cooking!

Thank you!

Thank you for embarking on this journey toward better health through nutritious and delicious low-cholesterol meals. Your dedication to improving your well-being is reflected in the completion of this cookbook, and we are privileged to have played a role in your journey.

We trust these recipes will inspire you to create meals that not only satisfy your taste buds but also enhance a heart-healthy lifestyle. Every recipe has been thoughtfully prepared with natural ingredients that are both tasty and helpful in maintaining good cholesterol levels.

May God heal and grant you sound health as you continue enjoying these foods. My wish is that through these dishes, you will experience increased energy, vitality, and overall wellness.

<u>If this cookbook has helped you, please consider writing an honest review. Your feedback is invaluable as it enables other people to discover the advantages of low-cholesterol diets. We are grateful for your support and for sharing your experiences.</u>

Thank you once again, and we wish you all the best on your journey to a healthier, happier life.

My sincere thanks,
Dr Debra Lincoln.

Printed in Great Britain
by Amazon